The Human Side of Medicine

The Human Side of Medicine

Three Generations of Family Physicians Share Their Stories

Joel Merenstein, MD

Jonathan Han, MD

Jennifer Middleton, MD, MPH

Foreword by Jack Coulehan, MD, MPH

Afterword by Paul Gross, MD

We would like to acknowledge the following publishers for permission to reprint the following material:

"The Family Doctor: A Tribute" is reprinted with permission from *The Journal of Family Practice* 39, no. 2 (1994): 111–122.

"My First Patient" is reprinted with permission from *The Journal of Family Practice* 51, no. 9 (2002).

"I Want to Die" is reprinted with permission from *Family Medicine* 40, no. 7 (2008): 512–13.

"Unknown Heroes" is reprinted with permission from *Family Medicine* 45, no. 2 (2013): 128–29.

(Continued on page 242)

First printing 2016
Printed in the United States of America

20 19 18 17 16 15   1 2 3 4 5

ISBN-13: 978-1523856800
ISBN-10: 1523856807

*We dedicate this book to our colleagues and patients,
whose lives make up the stories that inspire us all.*

*Joel: To Nancy Merenstein, who has shared
all my life stories and has always been my first reader,
advocate, critic, and supporter for all I have written
and all I have done during our sixty years together,
and to my children and grandchildren who make
our lives worthwhile and meaningful.*

*Jon: To my parents, Dorothy Sang Ye and James Sun
Nam Han, and to Marilyn, David, and Grace.*

*Jen: To my husband, Dave,
my parents, and my SPF.*

Contents

vii   Foreword by Jack Coulehan, MD, MPH

xi   Introduction: The Human Side of Medicine

1   **Part 1: Joel Merenstein, MD**

5   The Family Doctor—A Tribute

9   My First Patient

12   I Want to Die

16   My Most Unforgettable Patient

20   Remembering Mr. Palombo

25   Unknown Heroes

30   Malpractice?

34   The Doctor-Patient Relationship I

38   The Doctor-Patient Relationship II

43   The Doctor-Patient Relationship III

50   A Preceptor's Story

53   What Will I Do Without You?

57   The Family Doctor: A View from Retirement

63   **Part 2: Jonathan Han, MD**

67   The Kindest Insult

70   Welcome to the Arctic Circle

73   Malignant Neglect

80   Procedure Note

88   Serious Side Effects

91   Passing the Torch: A Day in the Life of an Attending Physician

101   Calculating Caring

110   Steep Sledding

113   Minutes

115   Bereavement

117   In Line at the Maine Clam House

121   Part 3: Jennifer Middleton, MD, MPH

125   Today I'm Grieving a Physician Suicide

131   Fallibility/Forgiveness

138   Our Family Doctor

142   A Eulogy to My Former Self

Selected Posts from "The Singing Pen of Doctor Jen" Blog

146   A Paper Cut in a Digital World

148   What Ever Happened to "Doctor"?

150   White Coats

152   Googling "Family Medicine": Who's Defining Us?

153   The Same Look

157   It's About the Run

159   My BHAG for Family Medicine

162   The Stack

164   Burnout and Redemption

167   Recipe for a Vital Primary Care Workforce

173   Part 4: Discussions Among the Writers

173   Introduction by Beth Merenstein, PhD

186   Why Do We Write?

209   Making Mistakes and the Dark Side of Medicine

222   Transitions: Saying Good-bye

227   Conclusion

229   Afterword by Paul Gross, MD

232   Acknowledgments

237   Contributors

239   Resources

242   Permissions

245   Author Bios

Foreword

By Jack Coulehan, MD, MPH

The two teachers I most remember in medical school were diametric opposites. One was the chief of medicine, known throughout the academic world for fire-breathing rapacity, as well as unparalleled clinical knowledge. He could fit every clinical fact precisely into a coherent pattern that he called the "whole person." In fact, the Chief's signature claim was that a good internist always treats the whole person—not a lab value, not a kidney, not a GU system, but the complete human being. Yet the man was a martinet who terrorized medical students, residents, and nursing staff alike with his steely gaze and unpredictable tantrums.

The second teacher was an elderly psychiatrist who met with third-year students in small groups on their psychiatry clerkships. He was a rumpled, heavy-set man with a cigarette generally hanging from his lips. Though a psychoanalyst of great repute, to us students he seemed disorganized and hopeless as a teacher. We were interested in learning specifics about how to diagnose endogenous depression, while he spent the whole hour telling us fascinating but seemingly irrelevant stories about patients. No one ever considered skipping a class when the chief of medicine taught, but we looked for any excuse to get out of those psychiatric seminars.

It took me a while to understand the importance of the chain-smoking psychiatrist's lessons. For him, the art of healing was grounded in stories and relationships. The "whole person" was far more than the totality of complex interacting organ systems that make up a human being. In later life, I realized that in a paradoxical way the chief of medicine had also taught me the value of narrative: I've often told students and residents the story of his powerful emotional impact on me, and I've written essays in which he plays an important role in my professional formation.

I've learned to think of my life in medical practice as a vast network of relationships and to see each relationship as a series of stories. Witness the vignettes of my two teachers that came to mind as I reflected on *The Human Side of Medicine*. This book was a delight for me not only because its three authors adopt a perspective similar to mine in sharing their stories and personal reflections as family physicians, but because they embed two additional dimensions that make their volume unusually perceptive and perhaps unique.

One particular genius of this collection lies in its extension of the narrative across three professional generations, from Joel Merenstein's stories of practice near the very inception of family medicine as a distinct specialty in the 1960s to Jennifer Middleton's use of electronic medical records and a personal blog well into the twenty-first century. The three physicians model a multi-generational family as they swap stories and share their reflections on personal and professional challenges.

The other exciting dimension is the "meta" element to their conversation, especially in the book's final section, where they comment on common themes they write about and on the process of translating clinical experiences into published narratives. What leads a physician to write about his or her experience? Why? Does writing about patients enhance or impair the art of healing? Here the authors reveal their wisdom and wit, as well as their passion for practicing family medicine.

There have been extraordinarily rapid changes in medicine over the time period represented in *The Human Side of Medicine*. The specialty itself has grown from infancy to maturity against a cultural background that was becoming progressively more specialized, complex, and technologically-oriented. Likewise, the economics and patterns of medical practice have changed dramatically. A common feature of all these changes is fragmentation and distancing: more distance between patient and physician, less continuity of care. This is a situation that leaves patients dissatisfied and often leads physicians to burnout and the loss of their passion for medicine.

But all is not lost. Far from it. There is a tough, committed cohort of patient-centered physicians in our midst. *The Human Side of Medicine* demonstrates that the art of healing is alive and well.

Introduction:
The Human Side
of Medicine

As the noted playwright, author, and physician Anton Chekhov lay dying of tuberculosis at a spa in Germany, a young doctor was called to attend him in his last moments. Instead of ordering tests or invoking other futile measures, the doctor sent for a glass of champagne. Sipping the sparkling wine, Chekhov commented, "It's a long time since I drank champagne." He then finished the glass, turned onto his side, and quietly stopped breathing.

The story of Chekhov's death has been dramatically told and retold, and it is captivating on many levels. How stressful it must have been to be the young doctor who had been called to attend to the famous writer in his last moments; what equanimity and wisdom it took for the doctor to prescribe one last medicine—a glass of champagne and his attending presence. The story captures much of what we long to experience as physicians and patients: to be treated with wisdom and grace in the most trying moments.

The interest in balancing humanity and science in medical practice—and the mindfulness of the practitioner about doing so—is not new. Hippocrates, writing around 400 BCE, noted that "it is often more important which patient has the disease than what disease the patient has." His emphasis on the patient as an individual is notable despite the fact that little was known about diseases and their etiology back then.

Introduction

William Osler, one of the most respected clinicians of all time, emphasized the importance of the doctor-patient relationship and getting the diagnosis from the patient himself. Instead of relying solely on examination skills and laboratory tests, he urged his students to "listen to the patient, and he will tell you what is wrong with him."

As medical knowledge advanced, physicians were increasingly able to give precise scientific explanations for their patients' ailments. Some doctors began to worry that the human side of medicine was being lost. In 1927, Francis Weld Peabody gave an address titled "The Care of the Patient," in which he reminded the graduating class of Harvard Medical School of the importance of respecting patients' humanity. Peabody noted that older doctors thought younger doctors knew a lot about the science of medicine but "didn't know how to take care of patients." Peabody ended his presentation with this statement: "The essence of the care of the patient is in caring for the patient."

Over the past fifty years, George L. Engel, MD, developed the *biopsychosocial* model, which explained illness as involving the biological, psychological, and social aspects of a person's life. More recently, physician Rita Charon has championed the *narrative* model, which focuses on illness as a story the patient tells. Other modern terms such as *patient-oriented medical care* and *patient-centered decision making* emphasize the nontechnical, personal part of the illness experience.

Physicians have been writing about their interest in this balance of humanity and science for centuries. William Carlos Williams and the aforementioned Anton Chekov are among the most famous doctors who wrote poignantly about their work. Prominent doctor-writers today include Jack Coulehan, Jerome Groopman, Sherwin B. Nuland, Atul Gawande, Perri Klass, and Abraham Verghese. Today, many medical journals include stories written by doctors alongside research articles. These stories importantly remind us of our patients'—and our own—shared humanity, but these stories have additional value beyond evoking emotion. In his book *The Call of Stories*, Robert Coles recalls conversations he had with "Doc Williams," who told him, "We have to pay the closest attention to what we say. What patients say tells us what is happening to us—what we are thinking, and what may be wrong with us . . . . Their story, yours, mine—it's what we all carry with us on this trip we take, and we owe it to each other to respect our stories and learn from them."

Cole reminds us that "the further one climbs the ladder of medical education, the less time one has for relaxed, storytelling reflection. And patients' health may be jeopardized because of it: patients' true concerns and complaints may be overlooked." Respecting the story—and the role of doctor and patient in it—not only facilitates compassionate care but can also ensure that the physician makes the correct diagnosis.

Even in research, we communicate with stories. In family medicine, we often use *qualitative research*, which focuses on meaning, not empirical facts. For example, the landmark Diabetes Control and Complication (DCCT) study reported the benefits of tight control of blood glucose and its relationship to cardiovascular and other complications in diabetic patients. But surprisingly, tight control of blood sugar was not associated with improvements in cardiovascular health but was correlated with an increase in potentially fatal low-blood-sugar (hypoglycemia) events. In a concurrent study published in the *Journal of General Internal Medicine*, researchers asked people with diabetes to tell their stories of hypoglycemia, yielding stories of fear and anxiety. So while the statistics tell us about the disease process, the stories tell us about the people. When physicians listen to their patients' stories, it helps physicians and patients make better decisions about improving patients' health.

Walling and Shapiro wrote in *Family Medicine*, "Reflective capacity has been identified as a core clinical competency that allows physicians to be attentive, curious, self-aware, and willing to recognize and correct errors. Reflective writing uses a personal story to enhance self-awareness and personal growth." Borkan and coeditors note in their book *Patients and Doctors* that storytelling is a basic element of human life. Medicine has a long history with storytelling, which was once the primary medium of medical knowledge since it was through stories that doctors and patients gave clinical accounts. The centrality of stories in medicine was lost with the growth of scientific knowledge and technology, but it is being rejuvenated by family medicine practitioners and other primary care specialists.

About the Authors

There are many anthologies of physicians' writings about their patients' experiences with illness and recovery. Our book contains stories examining the relationship between doctors and patients. All three of us hold the power of stories in high regard. Stories are not totally true or factual. They are recollections—partial memories imbued with the physician's beliefs, morals, and goals. These stories tell us not just the experience of a particular individual with a particular interest but also about that particular doctor and that doctor's experience.

Our book is also more than a collection of stories. It includes extended conversations among ourselves as teachers and practitioners of family medicine across the generations. Joel Merenstein retired from practice ten years ago after forty-two years of practice in the same location, Jonathan Han has practiced in several cities and is in the middle of his career, and Jennifer Middleton is in her eighth year of practice in an academic position. Our conversations add multigenerational perspective about balancing humanity and science in family medicine.

While our generational differences are evident throughout this book (and analyzed by contributor Beth Merenstein, PhD, in the introduction to Part 4), our similarities are hopefully even more so. We all value the importance of building longitudinal relationships with patients and families. We each find meaning in putting pen to paper (or fingers to keyboard) and cherish the opportunity to share our reflections on this peculiar life we have chosen. We all acknowledge the supreme privilege of witnessing our patients' struggles and triumphs.

Writing requires careful observation and intentional introspection, traits that the best physicians we know have in common. We hope that being physicians has made us better writers and that being writers has made us better physicians.

How to Read This Book

Our book is arranged into four sections. The first three parts contain the writings of each of the three authors: first Joel, then Jon, and last, Jen. The fourth section has transcripts of conversations that Joel, Jon, and Jen had from 2008 to 2012 about some of the stories in this book.

The commentaries are in a separate section after the stories because we want you, the reader, to form your own ideas and determine what message each story conveys to you. In the transcripts, each author is identified in capital letters ("JOEL," "JON," or "JEN"). Each author's section is also headed by a transcribed comment from the author.

Most of the pieces in the authors' sections have been previously published, and those references are in the reprint permissions. Additionally, we have included a resource section on where to publish stories like ours, for writers of all generations who wish to publish their own stories.

Part 1
Joel Merenstein, MD

I am Joel Merenstein, the oldest of the three authors who contributed to this book. I was in practice for forty-two years before I retired, and I practiced in a single specialty group in the same location for those forty-two years.

These stories probably tell more about me than my patients—or maybe they're about "us," the doctor and patient together. Francis Weld Peabody, in his famous address to the graduating class of Harvard Medical School in 1927, noted that the essence of the care of the patient is in caring for the patient. Michael Balint, in training general practitioners to care for their most difficult patients, discovered that the practitioner prescribing himself was the most important therapeutic tool the practitioner had. One might think that in these days of high technology—which brings the ability to diagnose more completely and treat more appropriately and effectively—that high touch is not necessary. But in fact, it is more necessary than ever as more patients long for an earlier time when doctors cared more and gave more, even though—or perhaps because—they could do less.

The stories here are but a small portion of the stories I lived with my patients. They are not the best, the most important, or even those that have affected me the most. They are stories that caught my eye or mind at a time when I wanted to share, had the time and energy to write, and felt that sharing would benefit the patient or family or at least do no harm. My job was to care for patients. Telling our story came later, often much later, and thus could not influence my care, decision making, or advice.

Although I always cared, I wasn't always very adept at the science of the art of medicine. There is a science to it, or at least there are some right and wrong ways to listen and talk to patients; to hear what they say and what they don't say; to recognize their nonverbal clues and your nonverbal communications; and to apply your need to help to their needs and wants. I still remember that as an intern and young doctor, I did and said some things that were not helpful to my patients; at times I was even callous and unconsciously uncaring. I won't share those stories here. It's enough to confess that they happened and remain a part of my memory forever. Instead of telling those stories, I have tried to tell stories that convey my failings and humanness as well as my strengths. By admitting to my early weaknesses, I don't mean to imply any new approximation of perfection, but I do think by the time I retired I really knew how to care for patients and teach those ways of caring to future doctors.

When I graduated medical school in 1960, there was no family practice specialty, and the number of general practitioners was rapidly decreasing. After a one-year rotating internship, I spent two years as a general medical officer in the air force. My experience in the service proved the adage that you can learn a lot of facts but you don't learn how to care for patients until the first year or two of practice. However, like many practitioners, when I left the service and joined an older practitioner in a suburban practice, I soon felt overtrained in many areas, undertrained in others, and generally dissatisfied. That's because I didn't know then what I know now: medical practice becomes fascinating and challenging if one focuses on the *patient* and his or her illness, not on the disease itself.

But at the time, I thought the solution was to leave medical practice and do other things. Instead, I cut down on practice hours and began to branch out. I sought out one of my medical school professors and began my first research project. More importantly, I started Balint training, which focuses on the doctor-patient relationship and how to deal with difficult patients. It gave me a new way of thinking about all my patients and about myself as a doctor.

The Balint seminars were organized and run by three outstanding psychiatrists—Rex Pittenger, Ralph Zabarenko, and Ralph Coppolla—who were interested in the care of patients by primary care physicians. After three years of group seminars, I proposed more direct training. Ralph Zabarenko agreed and joined me for the first hour of evening office hours every Thursday for the next year. We published our experience in the *Journal of the American Medical Association*, but the effect of that experience on me and how I practiced was much more important.

Subsequently, I became part-time faculty at the medical school and started working with new colleagues on two new courses: "Introduction to Patient Care" and "Patient Interviewing." I moved to a community hospital, the University of Pittsburgh Medical Center St. Margaret, where I started a fellowship to train family doctors to be teachers and faculty in family medicine. I also began a seminar series for medical students called "The Human Side of Medicine," and I did direct observation of residents and gave them feedback on their care of patients.

Since retiring from practice, I have continued some of my faculty activities and begun teaching or facilitating discussion groups on "The Human Side of Medicine" for Osher Lifelong Learning programs. I have mostly used the published stories of others as a basis for these activities, but in this book I've included some of my own stories as well.

As a result of my interest in stories and the doctor-patient relationship, I was intrigued by the number of letters and notes I received over the years from patients. I contacted my daughter, a sociologist and college professor, and together we analyzed these messages. Seven themes were evident in regard to what patients appreciated in their relationship with their family doctor: "being there," caring, medical expertise, personal characteristics, multiple roles/anything goes, family, and continuity. These findings confirmed the results of theoretical surveys and other studies, but they were based on real long-term relationships. These attitudes and comments, published in the *Journal of the American Board of Family Medicine*, tell a story of one doctor and multiple relationships. The stories here are more detailed and more personal, but for the most part, they contain the same themes.

My stories collected here show my progress from learning from an older experienced family physician to recognizing special patients with special ideas to sharing the experiences and feelings of both doctor and patient involved in this special relationship to retiring and leaving.

It's my biography, but you may have to look hard to see it.

The Family Doctor: A Tribute

While planning for a meeting with neighborhood leaders to develop more community outreach programs for our residency, I began to think about my original partner. He was a part of our community in a way that I never was. He opened his office in Renton, Pennsylvania, a small mining town, and lived behind the office. When he went off to serve in World War II, the community waited for him—not that they had any choice in those days. Within a few years after the war, he opened a second office in an adjacent rural community and moved his living quarters out of the office into a comfortable home a few hundred feet away. By the time I joined him, he had a second home, where he farmed. He delivered most of the young people in both communities and was the only doctor for those communities and the multiple small suburban areas that defined the 1950s. Some forty years later, I am trying to involve our residents with the urban neighborhoods we serve in a way that was natural to Dr. Waite.

I always called him "Doctor Waite," even after twenty years of practicing together, although people who didn't know him as well or as long called him by his first name, Knighton. Maybe it was because that was how he saw himself. He wasn't a formal person, often wearing his lumberjack-plaid shirts in the office and sounding very much like his neighbors in his language and choice of topics. He called most the patients by their first name and always called me Joel. But even on social occasions or at professional meetings with other physicians, I would hear him introduce himself as "Doctor Waite." I think it must relate to what another colleague recently told me about trying to adjust to retirement: "You know, nobody has called me 'doctor' in three weeks."

When I joined Dr. Waite in practice, I had just completed my internship and two years in the air force. It was not the practice I envisioned. I had never ventured far from the city and had expected to practice there, but the city was filling up with specialists, and I had opted for general practice. Dr. Waite had always been a country boy and often complained that he had settled in Renton to get away from the city, and now the city had followed him out. Many of the old-timers in the practice, including Mrs. Waite, who worked as a receptionist, felt the same way. All the office staff lived nearby and knew all of the patients and their families, if indeed they weren't related to them.

For the first few years, we maintained his practice pattern: hospital rounds early in the morning, an urgent house call on the way to the office, morning hours without appointments followed by scheduled house calls, a short break, and then afternoon office hours. We would each be in the office two evenings a week. I had no desire to do OB. He said he had done it all those years by himself so it wouldn't be any problem to keep doing it. Besides, he felt there was something special about delivering several generations of the same family. I had some sense of this years later, when I had established a special closeness to some families and they asked why I couldn't deliver their next child. He never got into the debate about whether family doctors should deliver babies. For him, it was just a natural part of caring for families.

We agreed on adding some new equipment to the practice. We bought a small incubator and started doing throat cultures, but I'm not sure he ever really trusted them against his clinical judgment. Now, when I discuss the sensitivity and specificity of throat cultures and rapid strep tests with residents, I wonder about the importance of this precision. I want to practice and teach scientific, rational medicine, but I also want to remember the power of the doctor-patient relationship. Was it so bad to give a shot of penicillin strictly on a clinical impression that included time for a cup of coffee and a little chat?

It wasn't long after I joined the practice that I began to discover and pursue my interest in teaching and research. I was quick to complain to him about all the time these activities were taking as a way of bragging about my achievements. He, meanwhile, continued quietly being part of the community. He served on the boards and several committees of the church and the bank and was active in Kiwanis, but it was the day-to-day informal involvement that really made him part of the community.

He had two homes within minutes of each other. One was in the coal mining town where he started practicing. He was the doctor for the coal company, yet the miners also chose him for their family doctor and never doubted his fairness to them or the company. He would treat their injuries and their infections and help them apply for their black lung benefits. There was never a disagreement about whether an injury was work related or when it was time to return to work.

We switched office hours to an appointment schedule, but that didn't stop people from dropping by his office or home. On the farm, they would stop by to exchange produce or ideas for increasing the crops and ask, "What do you think this is, Doc?" He didn't need a beeper. He was always there. He probably set as many fractures in the field as he did in the office.

Of course, he saw more patients in their homes than in his own. We made regular home visits each day between morning and afternoon hours. The only indication was that someone wanted one. You don't need to take much of a social history when you live with people and visit the sick in their homes. It's possible on those home visits to diagnose acute cholecystitis with an unusual presentation when you recall the patient's mother and grandmother presented the same way. Cost-effective analysis isn't needed either. When you make daily house calls, you say to those who can't afford to pay, "The man's sick and needs to be seen. Don't worry about paying for it."

It's been thirty years since I joined Dr. Waite and he carried in my boxes of books, telling me, correctly, that they were too heavy for me. He was a big, strong man. His scrapbook contained pictures of his college career as a star end on the football team, although he never talked about it or his experiences in World War II. He was a man of the present, not the past; a doer and not a complainer. In the summer, he would bring vegetables from the farm for everyone in the office, and in the winter, chestnuts from his trees and wood for my fireplace that he had cut himself. When we ate at his place, everything was home grown, including the chicken, the fish from the pond, and the berries in the pie that Mrs. Waite baked.

By the time he retired, we had merged our practice with a multispecialty group that provided an internist, a pediatrician, and nurse practitioners to our one modern office adjacent to two shopping centers. He had not delivered a baby for several years, and I had a half-time teaching position. He would have liked to continue practicing part-time, but the group decided it wasn't economically feasible to pay malpractice premiums and other costs for a limited office practice. He continued to work on the farm, recovered from several illnesses, and then died suddenly at home from complications following surgery.

I feel now about Dr. Waite as Mark Twain expressed about his father: "I left home at eighteen and came back at twenty-five; it's amazing how much the old man learned while I was gone." It has taken the years apart for me to realize how much Dr. Waite knew and taught me. Today, as I prepare to meet with our residents and the representatives of the communities we serve, I wish he were here. We're trying to develop community outreach for our residency and I'm supposed to talk about being a family doctor in the community. "Well, Knighton, what do you think I should say?"

Dedicated to the memory of
Knighton Van Buren Waite, MD (1911–1986)

My First Patient

"I remember the first time I saw you. I thought I was pregnant. You looked like a sixteen-year-old kid and you were going to examine me!"

Sharon* says that happened thirty-five years ago. I don't remember the incident. She is still my patient, and since then she and I have dealt with her breast cancer, depression, marital dysfunction, job frustration, and hypertension. Yet that first meeting remains vivid to her.

"You know, Doc Joel," said another patient, "I want to tell you a story before you inject my knee. Thirty years ago, you injected my thumb. If you can do as good a job with this knee as you did with that thumb when I first saw you, we'll be fine." He is the only patient who calls me "Doc Joel"; I appreciate this name as a token of affection. His memory of the injection of his thumb is clear; I don't remember it. Together we have coped with a recurrent skin rash, tuberculosis conversion with liver toxicity secondary to isoniazid, the death of his wife after a prolonged vigil in the intensive-care unit, and now osteoarthritis of his knee. Despite all that has happened, that initial contact remains important.

My patients often ask me whether I plan to retire—or more accurately, "You're not going to retire, Doctor, are you?" Many physicians in the latter part of their careers hear this all the time. Even our family practice residents are surprised at the intense feeling of loss that they and their patients feel after being together for only a few years. But there is an expression from my patients that I have not heard about from anyone else: "I think I was your first patient."

I have been practicing in the same community for some thirty-eight years. Lately, I've noticed that many of my patients want to talk about the time they first saw me. "How long have I been coming to see you, Doc?" they ask. "How long have we been together?" Some patients insist they have been seeing me longer than I have been in practice.

These statements are made with the pride of being part of something special. Robert McCall, the youngest seventy-eight-year-old I know, expressed this feeling graphically: "I believe I walked in the door of this building right behind you." So many people have made similar remarks that in retrospect, I must have seen a thousand patients that first week.

I am not in a rural practice where everyone is part of the same community. I live and practice in suburban communities. I am not active in civic, religious, social, or political activities. I would be proud to say I was the school doctor, a township board member, or a sponsor of a sports team, but I am not.

I have always enjoyed some of the trappings of being an old country doctor. Many of my patients grew up in the coal mining towns and farms that once filled the area around Pittsburgh where I work. That changed long ago as the city came to meet the country and coal gave way to cleaner fuels. I like going into the bank or restaurant and being recognized and called "Doc." It tickles me to be greeted with a smile or hug when I see someone who has changed doctors but still treasures our relationship. I like knowing my patients and their families and having them consider me almost a family member too.

But why is it so important to be the first? Now I often look at a patient's chart to see how long ago he or she made the first visit to my office. Sometimes I ask my longtime patients, "How long have we been together?" or "How long have you been coming here?" When patients claim to have been among my first, I feel elated. Maybe it's like remembering the beginning of a special relationship with someone you love. I still remember the first time I went out with my wife, which was before I met any of my patients. It *is* pleasant to recall that first time that led to so many years together.

My fantasy of specialness ended abruptly as I was making hospital rounds recently. Among my patients was a woman who had formerly gone to another family doctor. He had left a lot of disappointed patients when he moved away. As I was preparing to leave the room, she said, "If you see Dr. Coroso, tell him I said hello . . . I think I was his first patient."

All patients' names have been changed.

I Want to Die

"I want to die."

Frank made that simple declarative statement without anger or sadness when I entered his hospital room. He didn't look acutely ill and didn't appear to be suffering but went on.

"I've lived long enough. I can't take the pain and I want to die."

The vascular surgeon had readmitted him to the hospital the day before when he called with excruciating pain in his gangrenous left leg. On his previous admission and in the office he had declined the surgeon's recommendation that amputation would provide him the best quality of life, relieving his pain with the quickest rehabilitation. I agreed with the surgeon but also suggested hospice care as an alternative.

"Not yet," he had said.

Now I repeated the suggestion of hospice, saying that we would control his pain and keep him comfortable. He typically said little and would not explore his statement any further. He acknowledged that he had refused hospice on his last admission and didn't want to accept this alternative now.

His daughter from Florida, who had been quietly sitting by his bedside, informed me that he was already scheduled for the amputation. I spoke with his daughter-in-law, Terri, who provided most of his care. She and her family were also my patients. Terri agreed that Frank could make his own decisions. But what was that decision? He seemed clear in expressing his wish to die to me, but he had also understood the surgeon and had signed the consent form for surgery himself.

I actually felt the planned amputation was a good choice but also felt he had a right to refuse if he wanted to. Was he expressing his mixed feelings by agreeing with the surgeon and then telling me the opposite? Had we not controlled his pain and suffering well enough that he opted to come back to the hospital? Had he called the surgeon instead of me as a way of making a decision, or did he trust the surgeon more? If I had visited him at home rather than staying in touch by phone, would I have understood him better? Or maybe all of this was irrelevant. Ambivalence is what should be expected in these circumstances, and maybe saying "I want to die" and agreeing to the amputation were not contradictions at all.

I called the surgeon, who was in the hospital at that time. He reminded me that he had operated on Frank several times before and had also treated him medically for other problems. He would be happy to talk with Frank and his family again.

Was I expressing my own ambivalence by not joining this discussion? Did I just want the surgeon, as I knew he would, to convince him to have the surgery and absolve myself of responsibility? Or, at some level, did I understand that Frank could have it both ways—have the surgery and want to die at the same time.

Frank had a below -the-knee amputation of his left leg later that day. He had no complications, easily controlled pain, and recovered quickly. He was discharged in a few days to a rehab center to learn to walk with his newly fitted prosthesis. At the rehab center he was eating well, taking minimal pain medication, and beginning to walk. When I visited I pointed out how well he was doing and reminded him of what he had said when I first saw him at the hospital, feeling for sure that his desires had changed. "Well, what do you think now, Frank?" I said jovially and expectantly. Frank answered in the same matter-of-fact way that he did in the hospital: "I want to die."

I was surprised, not only questioning the decision to operate to which I had passively agreed, but also wondering, after all these years, why I didn't understand Frank's reasoning better. He offered little explanation despite my offer to try to understand what he was telling me. The rehab staff was unaware of these feelings and noted he was cooperative and even aggressive in his physical therapy. He expressed the same desire to his daughter-in-law, Terri, but never asked any of us to help him die.

Frank had always been a man of few words and no complaints.

On his first visit to me right after Thanksgiving in 1978, his history was brief and uncomplicated. He was fifty-nine and had worked in the coal mines since he was seventeen. He had never been sick but developed coldness and pain in his left foot and saw a podiatrist. The podiatrist referred him to me after finding decreased pulses and elevated blood sugar. Frank had quit smoking (for the first time) five years before but still drank a case and a half of beer in a week.

He quit drinking and his blood sugar was well controlled, but he never was able to return to work. The pain and coldness in his foot continued. Yet, he always said "I'm OK, Doc."

Life was not easy for Frank without work. He continued to meet his friends and limited himself to one to two "alcohol free" beers a day. His wife died suddenly and unexpectedly. As usual he adapted quietly and well. He settled into a routine. His son and daughter-in-law lived next door, and they spent a great deal of time together. He visited his daughter for a month or more to get away from the winter, first in Las Vegas and then, when she moved, in Florida. He always returned a little more animated, a little happier, and a little heavier. He saw me regularly but not frequently, on his own schedule.

Just before Christmas in 1990 he slipped on the ice and fell and broke his left ankle. He lay out in the cold and snow all night before a neighbor found him. He had the joint fused and the wound skin grafted. He had multiple complications and more surgery and spent months in the nursing home followed by home health with daily visits from the nurse. He sought out a variety of specialists, always fighting to get better and never giving up. I didn't really understand how he put up with the pain, the repeated hospitalizations, and the multiple surgeries, but he never complained, did what he was asked, and never said he wanted to die.

The following year he had a massive heart attack and heart failure and required an emergency high-risk bypass surgery. Again he had multiple complications but recovered well and never gave up. His recent reaction to the amputation and his attitude in the hospital and nursing home were thus new and different.

After he left the nursing home, I saw him in the office. He was able to walk down the hall using crutches and his prostheses. He didn't use the same words but told me that lots of his friends had died, there were few people around, and there really was no reason to live. He had refused antidepressants before or quit them too soon because "they didn't work" but reluctantly agreed to try again. Terri told me he only took them for a few days.

In January of 2005, he brought in his living will and made it clear he wanted nothing done even if he had a chance for recovery. The following year he was diagnosed with lung cancer with metastases, agreed to hospice care, told me and his family that he was ready, and died peacefully at home at age eighty-seven.

From this experience I learned that it is much easier to have a general discussion about patients' rights, shared decision making, and the right to die than it is to be sure you and your individual patient have done the right thing. How can we, as physicians, learn to accept ambivalence and recognize when what seems contradictory is really an appropriate decision? What is the proper role for the family, the surgeon, or the family doctor? Whose life is it, anyway? We may not always be right, but we can always care. Then we sometimes do the right thing without even knowing.

My Most Unforgettable Patient

When I was in junior high school, I always enjoyed reading the regular feature in *Reader's Digest* "My Most Unforgettable Character." In fact, I enjoyed the true stories in this column so much that I thought, *Someday, I'm going to write a story like that.* For a while, when I met someone particularly unusual or impressive, I would consider following up on this fantasy. But I didn't. Perhaps I forgot about the idea—or maybe I just didn't meet anyone interesting enough.

Then I met Bill Lacey.

Actually, I had met or at least seen him several times before, when I made house calls for his elderly mother-in-law. He was always in the house, but he said nothing to me and was hardly noticeable. But this meeting was different. This time, he was the patient, in the hospital to have prostate surgery. I was to examine him and be sure he was "medically cleared" for surgery.

Before entering his room, I learned from the nurse that he had already alienated his urologist and several of the urologist's colleagues. There were no other patients or visitors in the room. Bill was lying comfortably in his bed, smiling, content, and seemingly healthy. A large poster board stood on the sill, leaning against the window. The drawing on the board was more of a caricature, with a pronounced abdomen and a large arrow pointing close to the correct place and labeled "CUT HERE." As my attention was immediately pulled to the drawing, provoking a smile, he said, "The surgeon didn't think it was funny."

Over the next several decades, I would always find him and his cartoons funny, but besides the obvious jokes, I always wondered what else he was commenting on. In the early days of cholesterol awareness, he brought me a cartoon of two alcoholics (even though it was a pencil drawing, you knew they were drunks with ruddy cheeks and bulbous noses) sitting at a bar, drinks in front of them and the effects of prior drinks evident in their appearance. One was saying to the other, "You know, Albert, maybe we should go and get our cholesterol checked."

He would sometimes drop by my office and leave me a present with a note. Being a chocoholic and addicted to rich desserts, I wasn't greatly enthused by the bag of Zweibach crackers he left, but the note was worth it: "This is to celebrate Millard Fillmore's birthday. . . . By the way, who is Millard Fillmore?" The next visit I would ask about the gift and the note, but he wasn't into explanations. It was what it was.

He also gave me real presents with clearer meaning—but still without an explanation or a significant gift-giving occasion. He gave me a framed, perfectly executed pen drawing of the author Isaac Bashevis Singer, created at a recent speech by Singer, together with a quote from Singer in Bill's own calligraphy: "I will muddle through one way or another. I have developed my own theory: Not all maladies must be cured. Often the sickness tastes better than the remedy."

Singer was in his eighties when he said this. Bill was in his seventies but felt old since he'd been forced to retire. He had worked all of his life as a draftsman. Drawing, cartoons, and calligraphy were his hobbies. He loved working and having a place to go to every day. He found it funny but also inexplicable when a new thirtyish worker came in for his first day and put a sign above his desk that said, "2020 I'm outa' here." He seemed more disturbed by the lack of purpose in his life since retiring than his multiple illnesses.

He had mild diabetes, easily controlled with oral medication. He was thin and didn't need to change his diet. He was never much interested in food. He didn't ask about his lab tests or blood pressure readings, leaving those questions for his wife to ask. He was more interested in the books he read or perused when he hung out at the local library or bookstore. He gave me books to read that he had read several times, poems by Robert Service, and *Longitude*—a whole book about this aspect of geography. When I protested my lack of time to read, he insisted that I "keep them as long as you like, I don't need them."

He was not happy with the state of the world or the behavior of the human race. He was able to laugh about these observations and denied being depressed, "although my wife thinks I am." Prior to one visit, I got a note from his daughter that said:

> *My mom asked me to drop you a short note since you'll be seeing my dad later today. Lately he's been impossible! He's miserable twenty-four hours a day, but he claims nothing is wrong . . . He sits in a chair and stares into space.*
>
> *I guess there's not much you can do to help us, but when he comes in later and tells you he's just fine and has no complaints, picture in your mind one worn-out, frenzied wife and two exhausted, crazy daughters and know he's blatantly lying!*

Through the years, Bill had multiple small strokes and repeated falls, but when he came to the office he always said he was "just fine and had no complaints." When I told him about conversations with his wife and his daughters' reactions, he said, "I'm sure they're right"—and then went on to show me some drawings, discuss a book, or complain about the state of the world. He agreed to a trial of antidepressants more than once but didn't stay on them very long. No one noticed any difference in him.

Our visits were all the same and we both enjoyed them. We had lots to discuss as long as it wasn't his health, and I didn't offer any advice on what he should do. He had many interests; he knew a lot and was happy that I was willing to listen.

I retired from practice about a year and a half after he died. He was close to eighty-one. I still have some of the books he loaned me, including a poetry book I recently found that had some poems marked. One, by Service, struck me in its last lines as an appropriate message from Bill:

> I'd hate to be an animal, an insect or a fish.
> To be the least like bird or beast I've not the slightest wish.
> It's best, I find, to be resigned, and stick to Nature's plan:
> Content am I to live and die, just—Ordinary Man.

In my office at the residency where I still teach, I have a section of his work covering one wall. There's a cartoon and a drawing that his family gave me when I retired. The drawing shows a pitcher dropping the ball into the hands of the coach. The caption says, "So, you're finally stepping off the mound." I guess he wanted to be ready when the time came. I was pleased to know he was thinking of me—or perhaps it was a self-portrait and not meant for me at all.

There is also a sample of his calligraphy without a drawing. It's from Kafka's *A Country Doctor*: "To write prescriptions is easy, but to come to an understanding with people is hard."

We both understood that!

Remembering
Mr. Palombo

We met on May 17, 1965, when he first visited my office. His wife, who had been to see me before, was with him, as she would be for nearly every visit in the many years to come. They were Old World people in their dress, deference to the young doctor, modesty, and particularly their language. They spoke English with the melodious flavor of the Italian romance language they had grown up speaking.

We were at the same stage of life: married with young children, just starting our careers—he in the landscaping business and I as a family doctor. We would spend much time together as I tried to help him fight off his relentless diseases and he tried to make my small plot of land beautiful with stone walls, trees, bushes, and new grass. But the paths that brought us together were very different.

Mine was a pretty traditional American story. I grew up in a small city, met a wonderful girl in a teenage romance, fell in love, dated for four years, married, and started a family. I went to college after high school, medical school after college, and then did my internship—all in the same small city. I served in the peacetime air force within three hundred miles of home and later joined an established family doctor—less than two years before this visit when I met Ferdinand Palombo.

His path to our meeting was more of a story. Born in Italy in 1929, he served for eighteen months in the Italian army during World War II as a young teenager and worked in the army after the war. The first time he saw the woman who would become his wife, Pacifica, in the marketplace, he fell in love. When Pacifica went away to a college run by nuns to become a teacher, he started sending her beautiful letters. Knowing their story, the mailman who delivered Ferdinand's letters to her called them Romeo and Juliet.

Unfortunately, their families didn't get along because their fathers were business competitors, each owning a mill. Eventually they decided the only way to be together was to come to the United States so that they could marry and raise a family.

In remembrance of her parents, the Palombos' daughter Mary later wrote:

> The love between my mother and father was a true love. Their love did not have to be openly expressed for other eyes to see, for it was felt deep inside their hearts and souls. The first gift my father gave to my mother was a pen. It was a gold Aurora 88 pen he had purchased at a jewelry store for her birthday. My mother was away at school at the time, so he sent the pen by mail with white carnations— and a letter. In this letter, he asked her to write him using this gift so she would not forget him. He asked her to write of their love.
>
> When my mother's parents found out about the gift, they sent my aunt to go get the pen and give it back to its sender, along with a letter dictated by her father. When my mother wrote the letter, she began it with the words *Mon Amour* (My Love) written in French. She ended the letter *Amore vince tutto* (Love conquers all) in Latin. Those few words written in another language were the only words meant for my father, not the words written in Italian that all could understand.

Of course, I knew none of this as I sat taking a history about his headaches at this first visit. Over the years, I would see him often for headaches, low back pain, and a persistent cough. Then he developed diabetes, and though it was relatively easy to control, he suffered from multiple associated vascular problems. He had also had rheumatic fever when he was eleven. We thought he had no residual effects, but later, during coronary bypass surgery, the surgeons also replaced a diseased mitral valve caused by the rheumatic fever.

Now he had to have regular visits for the Coumadin therapy prescribed to protect him from clots from his artificial valve, as well as for his diabetes. As our visits became more medically complicated, he would wait to ask me questions about his health until he was sure my consultation with him was finished. I certainly didn't ask him about my lawn and trees until the visit was clearly ended.

Mr. Palombo came to my home twice a year with two or three men who would work all day trimming, pruning, replanting, cutting, and cleaning. In the beginning, he would work for a while with them. Once he felt comfortable leaving them, he'd give them instructions in Italian because they spoke no English, and he'd return at the end of the day to check on things. If I asked him a question in the office about a dying tree, the color of the lawn, or the lack of growth on the hillside, he would say, "I come and look"—and he always did.

After his wife had surgery for breast cancer, he stopped sending me bills. Despite my protestations, he wouldn't change this behavior. A psychologist friend of mine suggested that he might feel his wife would be OK if he took care of me. She rarely came for visits for herself to me or the surgeon, but even when she did, he never sent me another bill. She never had a recurrence or a complication.

In 1995, Mr. Palombo had a stroke, paralyzing his left side. He improved enough at the rehab center to walk with a cane; however, he became depressed and, with some minor variation, remained so, despite therapy, the rest of his life. His whole self-image had changed. He could no longer do the things that had made his business prosper: spending all day with his crews and every evening designing and pricing new jobs. His customers included estates in one of the wealthiest parts of town, as well as the state government, which accepted his bid to do all the new landscaping for the capitol in Harrisburg. His wife would say, "Telluh him he should feel lucky. We have our love and our family and he can still do a lot." But he would reply to me, as much as to his wife and himself, that he was useless or worthless.

The workers still came to my house twice a year, and he would come whenever I requested a lawn consultation just to get him active and out of his house. But I noticed that while the knowledge was still there, his enthusiasm was gone. His goal was to get back to normal; he didn't want to learn to live with his disabilities, and I wasn't successful in trying to change that attitude. Mrs. Palombo felt that this was really a good time because he wasn't working and they had more time to spend together than ever before. She was so proud of him. He was a successful businessman, a good father, a gentle and caring husband. They had never gone out much, happy to stay at home and be with each other.

In 2000, his last Christmas, he had his daughter buy a pen like the one he gave his wife in their Romeo and Juliet days. Mary said: "It was an Aurora pen. Once again my father wanted to give her a gift of a pen. A gift which carried the same meaning as the first one—the deepest meaning of love between two people."

Mr. Palombo died after forty-six days in the hospital in October 2001. We had known each other for thirty-six years.

I have now retired from my practice. My wife and I moved from our house to an apartment a few months after my retirement. I don't have a landscaper anymore. When I visited Mrs. Palombo in her home shortly after her husband died, she told me, "Now, young people don't have love like we had." We talked about family, good times, and difficult times.

When I was ready to leave, she said, "Doctoor, do me a favor." She had never, ever asked anything of me in the past other than to care for the husband she was so devoted to.

I said, "Certainly, Mrs. Palombo, if I can."

"Doan ever forget him, doctor. Doan ever forget him."

Unknown Heroes

Superheroes are found in comic books and cartoons. News-paper heroes usually are those that perform some clear, brave behavior that calls for attention. This is a story of the unknown heroes we work with every day, uncovered only through a clinical interaction with our co-worker's family.

John looked familiar to me when I first saw him on rounds, but I couldn't place him. As he stood by his father's hospital bed, I knew I had seen him around the hospital along with others who don't directly care for patients but make the hospital function: the human infrastructure. They wear their identifying uniforms in the same way that clinical people do, to separate us out by hierarchy and responsibility. The mail messengers and laundry workers wear casual street clothes; the maintenance men add a belt of tools; those cleaning the floors wear all blue. The men in dietary wear maroon baseball caps with the hospital's initials displayed in script above the brim. We often say hello and exchange some passing comment, but we never get to know each other.

Tim was the inpatient resident for the family health center service, and I had just started my two weeks as the teaching physician. Paul, our faculty psychiatrist, made rounds with the inpatient team once a week and joined us along with one of his trainees. When we entered the room, John was there with his mother, Mrs. Masters, waiting. John had come up from the cafeteria in his maroon uniform and stood next to his father's bed. John explained that his father had been ill off and on for ten years. Two years ago his father stopped drinking. He was then well until three weeks before admission, when he became jaundiced and wasted. Communication was difficult, as the patient was not only very ill but also deaf, and we would not have understood his sign language if he had had the energy to converse. The GI consultants had seen him soon after admission and had ordered lab and imaging studies. There was little doubt that he had late-stage alcoholic cirrhosis and very likely a complicating carcinoma of the liver. Tim had written "cancer" on a piece of paper and showed it to him. Although I'm sure John's father understood, he waved us off and conveyed that we needed to talk to his son while he rested. Tim, as the resident attending, explained the situation to John and asked him to consider the biopsy the consultants had recommended for his father.

With all of us gathered in the room, John said that he had already discussed this option with his parents, and they had decided against the biopsy. He then went on to tell his story. John was one of three children of deaf parents. When he was eight, his grandparents became aware that he could speak. They took him in and taught him and later sent him to military school to learn discipline, management, and responsibility. By age nine he had his own checkbook to pay the family bills and essentially managed the household.

As we talked, John's father sat up in bed, looked around without showing any sign of recognition, and then resumed his supine position. John leaned over to check on his mother, who seemed to convey messages in some mysterious way to John without any obvious form of language. John talked about hunting and other activities with his father and brother. The undisciplined fun and joy they shared was evident in his smile and in the animated way he told his stories.

When John said his mother had been the disciplinarian in the house, her smile confirmed that she knew what he had said and the pleasure she perceived at her success. I presume she read his lips, but I really don't know how she knew what he had said.

John had dropped out of high school in the 12th grade and left home "to get away from all of the family responsibilities." After he married and had three deaf sons of his own, he reunited his family with his parents and siblings so that he could take care of everyone. "What was I going to do? They needed me." His wife left two years ago, but now she was returning home with the children to be with John.

Recently another tragedy had struck the family. John's brother, Mark, was trying to rescue his dog from a lake near his home and drowned. John did not talk about grief or about losing his brother but instead about his responsibility and how, had he been there, he could have rescued his brother. John's mother, until then as attentive as the rest of us, began signing rapidly with an anxious look on her face. John interpreted for us. She admonished him that he would have drowned also in his rescue attempt and then she would have lost both sons.

This mother and son are alike and show they are used to carrying responsibility. They are built for it, small and not so much thin as trim, with small frames and anatomically clear muscle attachments without any fat. They stood or sat with military bearing, no slouch, no wavering, clearly conveying that they were where they belonged and knew what they had to do.

John continued his story. His sister, Jane, like their father, had a problem with alcohol. Paul, the psychiatrist just listening until now, acknowledged how difficult it would be to go through this again with his sister, then asked John if he or his mother had any questions. John said they knew what the facts were and what they had to do. Paul shook hands with John and his mother and thanked them. Others did the same as they filed out one by one. I hung back to be last. I anticipated that hug that I knew this brave, silent woman wanted to give. Her powerful arms reached up around my neck and told me not only how strong she was but also how thankful for our listening to their story and supporting her John.

We gathered at the nurses' station and talked about John as much as his father. The psychiatrists commented on getting some help for John, who couldn't be so tough forever. Tim said he would follow up with John but wondered what to expect and what to tell the family on discharge tomorrow. I told Tim that his patient could start bleeding and bleed out at any time but more likely would just fade into a coma and die quietly. That night he started bleeding, bled out, and died.

Over the next several months when I saw John in the hospital, I asked about him and his mother. He used to make excuses for not getting any counseling or would just say he was all right. He would say, "Thanks for asking." One time he told me his mother wasn't too good.

"How come, John?"

"Well my sister is back home and, you know, she's got the same problem as my father. I don't know if my mother can go through this again."

"What about you, John?"

"Oh, you know me, I'll be okay. I'm going to see if I can adopt her kids."

John happily showed me a picture of his whole family, including his sister's kids. He never did get the recommended counseling. John changed jobs a couple of years ago, now collecting laundry in the hospital without his maroon cap. He is always busy, never seeming to take a break, never complaining, and always smiling. We talk briefly. Occasionally he shows me a picture of his family. Last week he introduced me to his oldest son, who had just started working in the hospital. Chris looks more like John's mother than John but has John's energy and smile. John said, "He's deaf and doesn't talk." This may be true, but his son quickly demonstrated to me his grandmother's skill at conveying feelings without words. Chris may not know his father is a hero, but he was clearly proud to be working next to him in his hospital. Me too!

I'm sure there are more unknown heroes in our hospital that keep the hospital running while dealing with their complicated lives. I try now to be more friendly and supportive, but I don't probe into their personal lives. They are not my patients or my friends, but I hope they know that I care about them and respect them.

Malpractice?

"You let me down, doc, you let me down." Hank greeted me as I walked up the path to his home on this bright sunny day. It was not an easy decision to come to Hank's house to express my sympathy at the loss of his wife, Shirley. I always made some kind of contact when a patient died. It was not only helpful for the family but also helped me deal with my own sense of loss and sometimes a feeling of failure.

This was different. I had been out of town when Shirley died. My nurse, who had gone to the funeral home, told me that the family was very angry and blamed me. I knew I had to go, and though it was never easy, this would be particularly difficult. We shook hands and went into the house—where Hank's son and daughter, unsmiling, glared at me. I said I was sorry for their loss and asked if they had questions or anything they wanted to talk about. This was pretty much what I usually said, but now I was fearful I would not be able to tolerate their response.

Hank sat down on a footstool and I on another one close to him. Sue, his daughter, remained on the couch nearby, saying very little, while his son, Mark, stared at me venomously and said, "I've been telling them for years that they should change doctors." Hank added, "Maybe we were too close. Maybe it's not good to have the same doctor for over thirty years."

The rest of the visit went along these lines. I was not there to defend myself or make excuses but to pay my respects to Shirley and share my grief with a family I had known almost since I started practice. I said something like that and tried to respond to reasonable questions with reasonable answers.

Then Mark spoke again. "You should have found the aneurysm a long time ago; even when you did, you waited too long to call us." Where was Mark's anger coming from? I had seen him less than anyone else in the family. I had cared for him when he had an unusual, serious illness and was in the hospital a couple of years ago, but subsequently things had gone well, and although I had not seen him again since then, I was not aware of any problem. Certainly, his parents and sister never said anything on their many visits to the office. I had come to accept anger at me at the loss of a loved one, but his vehemence seemed unusual and even frightening.

Sue was a patient also, yet I mainly saw her when she brought in her children. She also took them to a pediatrician but expressed trust in my recommendations. Hank had had several serious illnesses, including an almost fatal pneumonia, in spite of which he had been coping well the past few years.

I saw Shirley most often. She had hypertension and arthritis, yet my major focus was to provide support for her anxieties and multiple worries and to enable her to quit smoking. Her last illness, however, seemed to worry everyone but her. She had abdominal pain and had lost weight. The weight loss wasn't unusual; she had lost and regained weight several times before as together we dealt with various stresses in her life. After several visits—with negative exams and normal blood tests—we agreed to get an ultrasound of her abdomen. I was afraid we would find the cancer she had always feared.

Instead, there was a large complex aortic aneurysm. The report sat on my desk for a few days while I tried to figure out how to tell her what we had found. I was especially concerned about the risky surgery that would be needed, knowing she would become anxious and depressed and maybe even panic. However, when I did talk to her, she was not as upset or as frightened as I had expected—either that or she simply didn't express her fears to me.

I called one of the vascular surgeons at our local hospital with a lot of experience with aneurysms, sent him the ultrasound report, and made an urgent appointment for Shirley. He called to say we needed to proceed with surgery but first needed additional imaging studies to better define the aneurysm. This would be a risky surgery but less so if the pictures enabled him to see better what he would be dealing with. I trusted his judgment, and the family and I accepted the plan.

He scheduled more X-ray studies; informed me, Shirley, and her family that this would be a very difficult operation with much danger; but said there were no other options. I spoke with her before I left for vacation, apologized that I wouldn't be there for her surgery, and assured her she was in good hands.

Two days before the scheduled date of surgery, the aneurysm ruptured. She had emergency surgery, but she never recovered and died a few days later. I did not hear about it until I returned and my nurse told me her story.

As difficult as that home visit was, I was still surprised to receive a letter from an attorney requesting Shirley's records. I had been in practice thirty-five years and had never been named in a malpractice suit. Then the previous year I had had two. I was not the primary defendant in either of these and was dropped from the suit when the primaries settled. Still, I was more sensitive to requests from lawyers, particularly if they came when most families were still in the grieving period.

I did not hear from the family, which only heightened my concerns. I began sleeping poorly, waking often, usually in the middle of an unremembered but horrible dream. I fretted and obsessed during my waking hours as well, whether at work or with my family. Then I remembered that Shirley had had a cardiac catheterization a few years ago. That should have shown an aneurysm if she's had it then, and the cardiologist would have called me. But what if he had not called and I had missed it on the report?

As I searched through volume one of her extensive chart, I was afraid to look and afraid not to look, worried that I would find that I had truly missed this serious diagnosis. There it was:

her coronary arteries were fine, but she had an aortic aneurysm. Now, not only was I going to be sued, but I was guilty! What would happen to me? How could I support my family or plan for the future? How could I have been so careless?

My sleeping became worse, the dreams now memorable and specific and even more horrible. I could not find pleasure in anything and could not concentrate on my patients' needs.

I'll tear the report out of the chart! I thought to myself. But of course, besides being stupid and of no use, that would be criminal. So I convinced myself that I had to at least go back and look at the report and consider what I could do.

After evening hours, once all the patients and staff had left, I pulled out that same volume one. There was the report. But there was no mention of an aneurysm! I slowed down and read again. I sat and thought, calmed myself, and read again. There was no aneurysm. I had somehow seen what I feared I would see.

There is a two-year statute of limitations on malpractice suits in Pennsylvania. I slept better and functioned better during the rest of those two years, but I always expected that accusing letter to come. It never did. When the last day of that two-year period came and went, I was shocked and exuberant.

But I felt sad and incomplete that I never saw anyone in that family again.

The Doctor-Patient Relationship I

Mary Ann and I had a long and intense relationship as patient and doctor. She was bright, resourceful, and determined. She had her own ideas about medical management and did not hesitate to share them with me. We usually disagreed—until she was dying.

Actually, for many years our conflicts centered around her role as mother rather than patient. I believe, and still do, that both the doctors' and the parents' responsibility for children should be to aid and encourage independence. Mary Ann believed in total protection and guidance. So many of her phone calls would start, "I know you think I'm an overprotective mother, but..."

Real crises were no problem for her. When the second of her four daughters had acute glomerulonephritis, she did not panic or become hysterical but remained calm, supportive, and caring. However, despite her daughter's complete recovery, Mary Ann would forever ask, "Shouldn't we check again to be sure her kidneys are still all right?"

As the girls grew older and less controllable, more of Mary Ann's questions and concerns focused on her own symptoms. Once again we had our disagreements. She was not a bothersome patient. In fact she would often wait weeks or months with a particular set of symptoms before calling or making an appointment; but when she did call or come in, she would always want more answers than I had, more explanations than I was capable of—and at the same time, she offered more suggestions than I knew how to handle.

She recognized some of her symptoms as depression and would start medication, only to discontinue the visits and the therapy before they could be effective. At other times she would request tests to evaluate her joint and muscle pains and then want to know why they were normal when she was so uncomfortable.

She never criticized me personally for the lack of answers but was often hard on herself. She came in for an urgent visit with severe ear pain. When I found a small furuncle in the external canal, she was upset that she had overacted and that the visit was unnecessary.

Whenever I recommended some referral or alternate form of therapy, she would counter, "That's not the answer," or "Do you really think that it will work?" When she finally agreed to see a rheumatology consultant, it seemed to be more to prove no one could diagnose her than to really get an answer. She was vindicated when the consultant could find nothing wrong.

Then a markedly elevated sedimentation rate was reported. This prompted an extensive hospital evaluation, but again no answers. Six weeks later she developed chills, fever, and lymph nodes so large that it was hardly necessary to biopsy them to diagnose her lymphoma.

As she began to do battle with the first of two oncology groups, the strengths of our relationship surfaced. In response to the oncologist's complaints, I noted that she had always been difficult. I told her and her husband that the oncologist should have been more open and informative. I was being truthful in both instances.

The second oncologist provided a little better communication but not much improvement or satisfaction. She failed to show any response at all to radiation or chemotherapy.

There was much for me to deal with, too: the lack of communication by the oncologist and their difficulty with her demands to know everything, a period of blaming her husband and then herself, and the oldest daughter's guilt feeling over her independence battles with her mother.

The oncologist reported there was nothing more he could offer. Mary Ann accepted this and prepared herself.

Then came the house calls. We talked about the home visits I made when the girls were younger and we were all just starting out. We reminisced and bantered, and then she nodded toward her husband and said, "You have to make him understand." So we stopped talking about the past and concentrated on the future.

Other home visits were to meet the visiting nurses and set up a regimen for pain medication and to see how things were going. There were no complaints and no disagreements. She made suggestions regarding adjustment of her medication and how the nurses might help. She was usually right, or at least she seemed to respond. There were no calls outside the regular visits until the end.

It was a cool but bright Sunday morning in March, and her husband called and asked if I could be there by noon. Her blood pressure had dropped, and they were afraid to give her the narcotic injection that was due then.

She was quiet but seemingly comfortable when I arrived. She said the priest had been there and given her the last rites and "everything was set." I asked one of the girls if perhaps they had last comments to discuss with their mother. She informed me her mother had already taken care of that.

Her daughters, her husband, and her sister were all around in the large master bedroom. We all talked together almost light-heartedly. She seemed to doze, and I said to the family, "Maybe she doesn't need the shot." We all laughed when she immediately admonished me, "You said the wrong thing!"

I gave the morphine and reminded her husband that the injections were not killing her but relieving her pain. I told her to put a good word in for me in heaven and said goodbye. At the front door I wanted to hug her husband but was only able to put my arm around his shoulder.

As I drove away I had a sense of loss but yet felt good that it went well. Then I had an uneasy feeling and pulled the car off the road and thought maybe it had gone well because we did things her way this time. She died at 6:00 a.m. the next day, quietly and peacefully at the age of 48.

The Doctor-Patient Relationship II

Edythe and I became good friends while her husband was dying. He had been to the office frequently until he finally developed the cancer he had always feared.

Edythe never came to the office. I only got to know her through his illness. We would talk in her kitchen after my visit with him. She never complained or asked what he and I had talked about. I would give her a brief update, which she accepted unemotionally but responded to with questions expressing her care and concern. We then would talk of our memories, plans, and common interests. I asked about their children and she about mine. As I left we would discuss how soon I should return as she offered her warm and inviting smile.

After he died we seldom saw each other, but she began sending me postcards. At first, they were just greetings for various seasons or holidays. Then she started to travel and the cards from across the country had comments about staying in touch and were signed, "Your friend." Sometimes there would be a hand-drawn picture of a smiling face. There was always a smile on my face when I read the brief notes.

Then, soon after I received her card from Ireland, she was admitted to my service at our community hospital. When I saw her, she wasn't very sick, had few complaints, and as always, was smiling. She stayed only a few days, but when the repeat X-rays in my office showed the pneumonia had persisted, she was readmitted to the hospital.

Our fears were confirmed. She had an obstructing carcinoma of the lung that appeared to be resectable. She agreed to transfer to the local university medical center.

Indeed, the lesion was resectable, but postoperatively she had a myocardial infarct followed by a bleeding ulcer. She recovered well, but as her days in the hospital increased, so did her complaints of vague chest and back pains. Finally, she was discharged, still smiling, but now with many complaints and discomforts. She couldn't sleep, couldn't lie down, and felt this constant tight band around her chest.

Her daughter, Patty, stayed with her for a few weeks and then returned to Florida. I spoke with her younger son, Kurt, often, as he had taken major responsibility for her care. He mentioned that prior to discharge from the medical center, the social workers and physicians agreed that just being in the hospital was depressing her. We wondered together if she was just unable to accept being sick after always being in good health and caring for others.

After several home visits, Bob, her oldest son, and Kurt brought her to the office. We agreed that she needed to be encouraged to begin the interaction with others that was always so nourishing for her. Perhaps coming to the office would be the first step. The visit was physically difficult for her as she told me, "I'd only do this for you." After the visit, the pains became worse. I suspected metastatic disease and reluctantly suggested another hospitalization. She was unhappy about more confinement but was so uncomfortable that she agreed.

Hospitals were not good for her. She arrested soon after admission. She recovered quickly, was extubated, and transferred out of the intensive care unit. Then her blood pressure started to drop and her urine output decreased. She showed minimal response to fluids and vasopressors. Although she had been returned to the unit, she refused any further interventions.

I spoke with Kurt the next morning. He said the doctor covering for me had spoken to them, and they had agreed to avoid any aggressive therapy. I was surprised to hear more anger than sympathy in my voice as I said, "It's her decision, not yours." I explained my position more calmly, wondered about my reaction, and went back to discuss the decision with her.

"That's enough," Edythe said. "I've been through enough. I'm tired and I don't want anything else done." There was no anger, only quiet determination.

I explained, bargained, and even pleaded, but she remained clear and decisive in her plan. "I waited for you to come, and now I want to wait for Patty. Then I'm going to heaven, and I don't want any interference."

I told her I would finish my rounds and be back. When I returned she admonished me, "I wanted to kiss you good-bye and you left."

"I told you I'd be back."

I lowered the side rails and removed the oxygen mask, and we kissed. She was warm and soft, with no sign, smell, or touch of death.

"Thanks for everything," she said.

"Thanks for being such a special person," I responded.

"You're my good friend," she said.

"That's why it's so hard to let you go."

Then her sister interjected, "There will be no one to send you postcards anymore."

The next day the ICU nurses told me she remained alert, responsive, and comfortable through most of the day and then just faded away. Patty had arrived from Florida. Her family was with her throughout the day.

Although I always call, write, or make a home visit after a death, I seldom go to the funeral home. When I do I suspect it's for some hidden need of my own, though a special closeness explains part of it. The parking lot was jammed as I arrived. As I approached the entrance I saw Kurt coming from the other direction. His bright clothes and jaunty walk contrasted with my dark blues.

When he saw me, his mother's smile on his face broke into a wide grin. We reached out to each other and he said, "I knew you'd be here." I was glad I had come.

We walked in together. I spotted Patty, who I had not seen since my last home visit. I told her I was glad she had made it in time. She said she was pleased also and told me how her mother had made it easy for them, as she always had. Others had come to her hospital room, and her mother had talked with them, but periodically she would call, "Kurt, Patty, Bob," and gather them around her for special comments and suggestions. "Don't forget to call Aunt X or Cousin Y," she told Patty while she continued with her special smile. She said good-bye a couple of times, and the last time Patty thought she "heard her talking to God."

As we spoke, Bob appeared on my right. We sensed a special closeness. Bob is an attorney and well acquainted with responsibility. Now we had gone through the death of both of his parents together. I still remember his call five years before at 6:30 in the morning. He simply said, "My father just passed away. Thanks for everything you did."

He and Patty then told me of those last few hours in the hospital. Their mother remained alert and smiling, and according to Bob, there was even some laugher. He noted how much harder it would have been if they had just received a call in the middle the night that she had died.

He said to me that it must be difficult dealing with suffering day in and day out. I always expect some comment like this and had thought about how I might answer. What I didn't anticipate were the tears that started to flow as I said that medicine is not all death and dying. Most days are just for simple routine problems.

I felt foolish with the tears running down my face as Edythe lay in the open coffin smiling while her children, with the gift of her smile on their faces, seemed so content. What particular feelings stimulated the tears, I don't know.

Afterwards, when I thought about it, I also remembered being perfectly calm and controlled greeting people at my brother's funeral a year earlier. As my closest cousin approached me, the tears had flowed in the same way. Then I recognized all the memories that contact reawakened. This time the feeling was the same, but the source wasn't so obvious.

As I collected myself, we began talking about the postcards she'd sent me. I asked Patty if she knew about the one I received from her from the medical center. On it she had drawn a picture of two buildings, labeling one as our community hospital and the larger one as the university medical center. Across the latter one she printed "Wish you were here." Bob said she received excellent care at the medical center but was feeling a lack of sensitivity and personal attention when she sent the card. I said I would miss her and her cards.

Patty looked heavenward and said, "Maybe she'll send you one from there." Maybe she will. Even without the postcards, though, I'll know she's smiling at all of us.

The Doctor–Patient Relationship III

He's my patient. I'm his doctor. There is no beginning.
There is no end.

—Ray Greco, *One Man's Practice*

I met Mary Nelson first. I won't pretend that I remember the specific event. My records state that it was the third of June, 1967. She was sixty-one years old and had recently moved to the Pittsburgh area from Illinois. Most likely it was a Thursday evening, because I do remember that I mostly saw her at night. Of course, back then I had evening hours twice a week.

Her initial problem list included hypertension, multiple somatic complaints, and chronic use of tranquilizers. The note from her doctor in Illinois was brief and to the point. She was a nervous woman whose blood pressure and symptoms were well controlled with minimal medication.

Her previous doctor had established a successful pattern, which I followed. I saw her every three to four months, checked her blood pressure, listened to her complaints, discussed some problems, and reviewed her prescriptions when necessary.

We spoke of various family difficulties, deaths of neighbors, conflicts with her son, and the financial problems. She noted repeatedly how dependent she was on her husband and how good he was to her and her children.

She had been coming to see me for over a year before Harold became my patient, at her request. As usual, he was in the waiting room during her visit. She said he needed help and would I talk with him.

43

Mr. Nelson was 10 years younger than his wife. He was short, about my height, but much more muscular. His cheeks were plethoric and his nose just suggested rosacea. He told me his story quickly but with detail. He was clearly upset when he couldn't hold back the tears.

He complained of dizziness and fatigue and somehow knew that it was related to his job promotion. He had gone from shop mechanic into the office and sales.

On subsequent weekly visits he talked about his increased responsibilities and the animosity of the other workers. He also, with tears, noted how he tried to help his stepchildren but never seemed to make much progress in their relationship.

After the fourth visit, I suggested he return in three to four weeks. It was nearly three years before he returned for me to remove a sebaceous cyst from his scalp. I knew he was doing well as I continued to see Mary every three months.

Two years later, he returned for a "checkup." His rosacea now required therapy, and we spoke of his complete break with his stepson.

I saw him two or three times for minor respiratory problems over the next several years. In April 1976, nearly nine years since they had first entered my practice, the first hospitalization occurred. Because of my teaching responsibilities I had temporarily given up my hospital practice at the local hospital. One of my associates treated Harold for his pneumonia, and Mary kept me informed. She again expressed her concern about what would happen to her if he were seriously ill.

He gave up his one-and-a-half packs of cigarettes a day and generally did well. A year later he had prostate surgery and tolerated it without difficulty. He was upset with the subsequent retrograde ejaculation and the lack of information from the urologist. I explained and reassured and chided myself for not doing so prior to the surgery.

By the following year (1978), his COPD had gotten worse. He had frequent acute bronchitis, required monthly visits to the office, and had another hospitalization. We discussed possible early retirement and applying for Social Security. He was upset with his insurance department, our billing office, the life insurance company, the red tape with Social Security, and the state of the world. I listened and helped where I could. We also discussed his concern about his wife's continued smoking.

His COPD was finally stable, although he required low-dose steroids most the time. He developed carpal tunnel and a cataract and tolerated both surgeries well (1981).

After the cataract surgery he complained to me of some persistent difficulty with his vision. But the real reason for the visit was to discuss some recent sexual dysfunction which really only required some explanation of the normal aging process.

Over the next six months, I saw him infrequently, and he was always well enough to complain about the government or some injustice in the world.

In April 1982, Mary was admitted to the hospital with severe shortness of breath. She showed poor response to therapy and had to be intubated. After a slow, gradual response she had a relapse and had to return to the ICU. She seemed to have no drive to get well. Her only request was to be allowed to continue smoking.

She did respond but relapsed a second time. She was alert enough to respond to questioning and requested not to be returned to the ICU and not to be intubated again. I discussed her request with Harold at her bedside.

I still remember our standing by her bed, searching each other's eyes for the right answer, and wondering what to do about our doubts. I asked her again. She had no doubts. Harold said it would be best to go along with her wishes. She died on April 29, 1982, at age seventy-five, after fifteen years as my patient.

We always knew how difficult it would be for her without him. We had never considered the opposite. He was devastated. "Hard to go on. Don't think I can make it. Can't get along with her."

He had developed some chest pains while she was in the hospital. Now, it was clear that it was angina. He was admitted to the hospital with coronary insufficiency, transferred to the university medical center, and had angioplasty of his right main coronary. It was four months since Mary's death.

Over the next year he was up and down. He remained on antidepressant medication. At times he was well enough to visit his stepdaughter in Chicago. Yet he also required several hospitalizations, once for pneumonia, once for recurrent angina.

While he was in the hospital, we consulted a psychiatrist regarding his persistent depression. He liked the psychiatrist but not his suggestion to move to a senior citizen apartment. "I'll never leave my home. I'll have to find some way to get through the night."

He was seen often, usually for his respiratory problems. He was always depressed. He exclaimed that he wanted to die but denied any suicidal thought or plans. I told him we needed to stay in close contact.

He had a couple more brief hospitalizations and was establishing a relationship with the cardiology and pulmonary consultants. He still had mostly bad nights and occasional bad days with the depression, but he functioned well and was proud of his new car, which he used to stay independent and take brief rides in the countryside.

As much for his benefit as for educational purposes, I invited Harold to join another widowed patient of mine in helping me with my annual presentation on the doctor-patient relationship to first-year medical students.

It was a nice day and we enjoyed our ride into the center city. The presentation went well as the two men talked about how they had each adjusted and who was the better independent homemaker.

There was friendly conversation as we rode back to my office. My hope that a mutually supportive relationship might develop seemed possible. But there was never any further contact between the two of them.

I saw Harold nearly once a month. It's interesting that when we first met, we were Mr. Nelson and Dr. Merenstein. During the years when my visits were mostly with his wife, he began calling me Joel. I reciprocated by calling him Harold. As he became more ill he addressed me as "Doc" or Doctor," and I continued with Harold, and that's the way we continued.

He seemed stable though persistently depressed until just before Christmas in 1985. He came to the office complaining of constipation and worsening depression. He then said he had something to show me. He told me he had bought the gun two days previously. He had come close but was unable to pull the trigger and then decided to call me.

I called the hospital and the psychiatrist to get him admitted and the police to pick up the gun. He saw the psychiatrist for two months after discharge and then refused to return although he continued his medications. He developed other medical problems including a colonic polyp and a compression fracture of his L1 vertebra, presumably secondary to the frequent use of steroids.

After a period of bed rest he improved again. He was well enough to visit his stepdaughter in Chicago and to attend his mother's eighty-eighth birthday celebration at her nursing home.

He bought himself a poodle and seemed happier than he had been in a long time. When he showed me the pictures and stated he hoped they'd have ten years together, I wondered why I hadn't thought about a pet as therapy.

Despite some setbacks—he couldn't take the dog to obedience school because he got too short of breath putting the dog through the required program, and his vision was failing because of macular degeneration—he remained active and upbeat. So I was surprised when he brought in his handwritten statement requesting no life support. He agreed to amend it to allow life support measures if there was a rational chance of recovery. After the nurse witnessed his statement, it became part of Volume III of his record.

Although he never required life support, his hospitalizations were increasing and his functional capacity decreasing. He had more angina, recent bronchitis, acute pulmonary emboli, another compression fracture, and a lacunar stroke.

I was his doctor in the hospital and the rehab center. I saw him every few weeks in the office and spoke frequently to the home health nurses. I never made a house call. That was a mistake.

He gradually told me about his increasingly close relationship with his neighbor, Mae. She and her husband always helped and cared for Harold, often bringing him to the office when he was too ill to drive. Mae brought him meals and invited him for dinner. Harold helped them also when he could.

Mae's husband then became severely ill with emphysema. I cared for him in the hospital, or rather I provided the medical care while Mae slept in her cot by his bed and cared for him. I received a nice note of appreciation after his death but didn't see Mae again until she began coming with Harold.

Their plans for marriage were almost canceled with another hospitalization for his angina. He stabilized in time to proceed with the ceremony. She took care of him, called him "Daddy," showed him affection, and managed his affairs while never taking away his sense of control.

He suffered so much he wanted to die. He was tired of the pain, the constant oxygen, the frequent hospitalizations, and the inability to do. Yet every visit there was a smile or a laugh and at least one off-color comment when Mae helped him get his pants back on.

I, unfairly, wanted him to keep trying. "If we can just get you over this next hurdle, I'm sure you're going to be okay for a while."

He either believed me, wanted to please me, or just didn't know how to give up.

His final hospitalization, he had a deep thrombophlebitis extending all the way into his iliac. He had chest pains, but we didn't look for pulmonary emboli. We did start Heparin and continued his meds.

On the day of admission he said, "This is it doctor, I can't go on anymore. Thanks for everything. I really appreciate it." He lost consciousness soon after admission. The nurses called about treating his arrhythmias. I talked to Mae a lot, but I didn't spend much time with him. He died October 29, 1990, at age seventy-four, after twenty-two years as my patient.

I never got a chance to tell him how I wanted to write this story to tell the world about this special relationship that doctor and patient sometimes have—that we had. I didn't cry until now, when I wrote this last sentence.

Mae and I talked on the phone. She brought some cookies and talked to the people in the office who knew Harold so well. Last week she came in for a checkup and pap test and brought some more cookies. "There is no beginning, there is no end."

A Preceptor's Story

It's been more than twenty years, but I still keep replaying the event, looking for another outcome. We all have these cases floating through our conscious minds, reminding us of our errors, the failures we couldn't prevent, or the worst ones—those for which we still don't know what we could have done differently. This is one of those, but it's not about a patient of mine. It's about one I precepted.

I had just started precepting residents on a regular basis. Most of my teaching experience until then had been with medical students. I had had my own practice for more than fifteen years, and I certainly wasn't a novice, but I wondered how my depth of knowledge compared to these residents. I knew I didn't compare to the rest of the faculty, who all seemed Oslerian in their knowledge. But I had done well so far, and I had always been comfortable with patients.

Ted was a particularly bright third-year resident who clearly wanted to learn more. When he asked a question, it wasn't to test the preceptor's knowledge or meet some requirement. He really wanted to know. Maybe I was the only preceptor available. Maybe he knew I was also leading Balint seminars since I had come to the program. Whatever the reason, he made it clear he needed help with this patient as he began presenting her to me. He had been seeing Gloria for several months now. Her complaint always remained the same: she had lower abdominal cramping pain that was severe at many times but was unpredictable in its appearance. She had no other symptoms. No nausea, vomiting, diarrhea, fever, or weight loss. He tried diet changes and symptomatic medications. Each time she came back with the same story, unchanged. She didn't seem depressed, and she wasn't demanding or complaining. She only wanted him to make the pain go away.

He knew they would be normal, but he ordered a variety of diagnostic tests anyway. They were indeed normal, but the pain persisted despite his reassuring her that everything was fine. He referred her to a gynecologist who found nothing and said it was functional. Now the patient was back to discuss the consultants' reports and see what could be done. Could I see her and make some suggestions?

She was sitting on the exam table with a gown on as we entered. Ted introduced me and then stood aside with the medical student who was working with him. I sat down in front but below her on the exam stool. I noted that I had heard about her story and that it must be frustrating and upsetting as well as painful. I asked if she could repeat briefly for me what had been going on these past few months. I followed her leads, which led me to ask about the relation of the pain to intercourse, which then led to questions about her marriage.

She was an attractive young woman, about twenty-five, and well composed until we treaded on this path. She began to cry after a few isolated tears slid down her cheek. She didn't interrupt her story, though, as she spoke of his demands and her disappointments. I handed her some tissues, patted her hand, and suggested that we had hit on something important that needed more exploration. I said that Ted and I would talk and that she should feel comfortable coming back so that he could continue to help her, and then I left. Ted later told me that she was fine when she left, that she had thanked him, and that she had said she would return.

Ted and I, with the medical student mostly just listening, talked about his patient and what had just happened. Why had she never spoken about these personal problems before, and were they truly related to her disabling symptoms? How do you convey to a patient that you are really ready to listen and that all topics are open for discussion? Why had she opened up to me and not him? He was a competent, knowledgeable doctor. He obviously cared for her and showed it. These were not advanced skills involving some complex procedure. We then talked about how to teach and learn these skills. Should we start a special course? Was role modeling as I had done the best way? We didn't come to any specific conclusions, but I felt good that I had been able to demonstrate for this excellent resident a way to deal with patients and address their real needs.

She never came back! I asked Ted about her for several weeks. He had called her several times. She never made an appointment. She never even called back. He was mildly disappointed. I was devastated. It was like, as a clinician, a patient dies after you were convinced you had made a brilliant diagnosis and implemented the perfect management plan. I wondered what I had I done wrong? Did I expose her or embarrass her? Did I take away her relationship with Ted? Why did I think I was so smart and so good a role model? Why does this experience stick with me, with the same feelings as from the death of one of my own patients?

Ted is now a residency director and an excellent teacher. I am confident that I'm a good preceptor, and I teach precepting skills to fellows—but I still wonder what happened to this patient, what I could have done differently, and what other preceptor stories like this are out there waiting to be told.

What Will I Do Without You?

"What will I do without you?" Mrs. M cried as she asked me if it was true that I was retiring. Although I have never raised the issue of my retirement with any of my patients, this question and others like it have cropped up. And, of course, as I get older the questions are more frequent and more reality based.

Mrs. M has been my patient and I her physician for thirty-five years. When I first saw her in March 1967, she was living with her husband and two daughters, with her parents nearby. All but her older daughter are now gone: her husband from metastatic colon cancer, her daughter at age nineteen from a perforated ulcer while taking prednisone for rheumatoid arthritis. Her parents died of heart disease: her father at eighty-eight, her mother at ninety. Mrs. M cared for all of them and they were all my patients.

She has easily controlled diabetes and hypertension and has survived knee surgery, cataracts, and breast cancer. We both still grieve for her daughter Jeannette, who died on my birthday in 1978. I'm not sure how Mrs. M knew it was my birthday, but we both always remember the association with that awful feeling of old grief. Over these years of loss and personal illness, she has never needed an antidepressant, counseling, or even much in the way of support. She comes in regularly for her chronic-care checkups but rarely requires a visit in between; she calls with problems or concerns even more rarely. She lives alone, travels frequently, and continues to care for and about others. Yet she wants to know what she will do without me if I retire.

Contemplating retirement is not something at which I have spent much time. Over the years when I get together with my two closest friends who live in California, we often speculate over dinner about the concept. The discussion is always vague and nonspecific. Now one has retired from his position as a tenured professor of education, and the other is seriously considering leaving his job as director of public relations at the post office. I also notice that more physicians are retiring earlier, fed up with the "new" health care system or just ready to do something else. So I contemplate retirement more often now, but my plans are still vague and nonspecific.

"What will I do without you?" John K has asked me this before, usually when he is recovering from some acute illness. Now complications of his long-standing diabetes are catching up with him and he wants to know that I will be there for him. He is still a big man—looking the part of the blacksmith he was for US Steel—who has always managed to work physically hard, climbing through trees and up chimneys even with angina or heart failure and always against my advice. He is now eighty-five and has been telling me for thirty-five years that he is weak and tired and won't live very long. With my urging he did quit smoking twenty years ago, and he does take his medicine as prescribed. Yet he eats as he wishes and takes unnecessary risks that I cannot influence. Though he has lived his life his way, he worries what he will do without me.

Contemplating retirement is something I guess I should be doing because so many people ask me about it now. My wife's cousin recently retired and moved to Florida. He asked me why I wasn't retiring and then proceeded to give me the answer himself: "I know all the answers: 'What would I do with my time? What else could I do that I would enjoy so much?'" These are indeed my usual responses, but I believe the real reasons go much deeper. I have been in practice in the same location for almost forty years. Many of my patients have been with me since my first years there. Some were patients of my original partner and have been in the practice longer than I have. As Michael Balint taught, the most powerful therapy I have to offer my patients is me, and I have tried that prescription as much as possible. The patient-physician relationship has sustained me and my patients and I hope contributed to our health and quality of life.

"What will I do without you?" Carol B is the last patient in my practice to have had rheumatic fever; she was twelve. She is now thirty-seven, works full time, no longer has a discernible heart murmur, has three kids, and is generally happy and healthy. The children have never had any serious illnesses and see me for routine checkups. There have been no major family crises and I have not been called upon to aid in any family decisions. They do fine on their own, but she still ponders what she will do without me.

Contemplating retirement was not much in my thoughts until recently, although I knew I wanted to quit when I still was at the top of my game. When I do consider retirement I get these ideas. I might make house calls to sit and talk with all of those people I never got to know in quite the detail that I would have liked. Of course, that's almost everyone, no matter how close we are or how much we have shared. I'd like to think my patients are concerned about my leaving because I'm a good and caring doctor, but I know it is much more complex than that. I have heard similar concerns expressed to most other physicians. When people say, "What will I do without you?" or "You can't retire until I die!" or "You're not going to retire, are you?" I know it's not just about me. Yet I have worried, *Will they be okay? Will the new doctor know as much or care as much? Am I deserting them for my own needs and pleasure?*

This past summer all of these questions were put into perspective. I underwent four-vessel coronary artery bypass surgery. The telephone calls, the cards, the questions at the office were a graphic portrayal of patients' feelings: they cared about me. One patient even showed up outside my hospital room door the day after my surgery. He had told my daughter he just wanted to be sure I was all right.

Being at home—recuperating—was depressing. I couldn't eat. I was exhausted all the time. But mostly I felt useless and unfocused. I returned to the office in three weeks even though I wasn't allowed to drive myself. My depression cleared then: whether it was the passage of time or getting back to my patients, I'll never really know. The caring was even more evident as I saw patients in the office once again. Those who knew about my surgery wanted to be sure I was taking care of myself. Those who hadn't known were shocked, but they expressed the same feelings.

But then I noticed something new and subtle over the next six weeks as I returned to my full schedule. Patients started to tell me how good my partners are:

"I saw Dr. Olbrich when you were out. He's really a nice guy and took care of me."

"That Stacey is so pretty and so nice. I know she'd prefer to be called Dr. Devine. Well, she was great, such a good listener. She also checked my cholesterol. It hadn't been done in awhile. I guess you and I forgot about it."

"Which doctor do you think I should see if you have to be out again?"

All of these portrayals were from people who were anxious to come back and see me, and I know they were partially, at least, to reassure me that I hadn't let them down. I was reassured and also pleased and proud of the group of family physicians with whom I practice. But I realized something else: These people will be okay when I am gone. They will get good medical care and be well taken care of. But what about me? I need that love and caring, that sense that I am important and will make a difference in someone's life.

No, my dear patients, when I retire, what will I do without you?

The Family Doctor:
A View from Retirement

Before I retired from clinical practice, I wrote *A Piece of My*
Mind entitled "What Will I Do Without You?" In it, I concluded it would be more difficult for me leaving my patients than it
would be for them. It has been! Granted, I really don't know
how well they are doing or how difficult the separation has been.
When I pay a social visit to them in the hospital, they seem happy and confident with their new doctor. My office notifies me
when one of my long-standing patients has died. I usually call the
spouse or other family members. They are appreciative and glad
to hear from me, but I can tell that I'm really not part of what is
happening. I am a concerned outsider.

Being in practice for forty-two years was like running a
marathon. Running at first seems easy and pleasant until you
hit that wall at ten miles, my son tells me. For me ten years of
practice was the equivalent. That's when you say, *I can't go
on, it's just too hard, what am I doing here?* If you decide not
to quit, and continue, the endorphins kick in. You feel a high
and know you could go on like this forever. Can life really be
this good?

And then, as the years pass by, you and your patients change
and you know the race is over. It's time to stop running. Yet, there
are many losses at giving up practice. After spending nearly a
lifetime as a doctor, it's hard to give up that identity. That's who
you are and have been. I saw the doctor-patient relationship as
"a covenant, not a contract," as Gayle Stephens described it, and

my role as a physician was to prescribe myself as my most potent therapy as taught by Michael Balint.[1]

David Loxtercamp[2] has written about "being there" as the prime service of the family doctor. But in retiring you are no longer there and you give up that faith and confidence your patients have had in you and the way that makes you feel special. What is unique about being a family doctor? I heard a British family doctor a few years ago define the family doctor as someone you can go to and talk about anything you want. To me the family doctor is someone who knows you, really knows you, in a way that no one else does; someone who is empathic not to walk in your moccasins but to become you, moccasins and all; someone who can cry with you at your loss not because they can appreciate your loss but because their loss is your loss too.

Many patients, when I retired, wanted to "go out to lunch" or in some way maintain our relationship. I have avoided this, saying that I thought it was important to develop a relationship with their new doctor. This was true and I really believed important, but I've come to believe it's not the most important reason. Lovers breaking up say, "But we can still be friends," even though they know that is impossible. They can neither give up the special feelings they have had nor the memories of those feelings, which will always be a relevant part of their lives. I have too much invested in these relationships to "just be friends."

Don't think that I haven't moved on. I am still teaching and doing research. My wife of fifty-two years and I travel and visit our children and grandchildren. I take and teach classes at a program for retired people. I have more free time and don't miss the constant responsibility or the agonizing over mistakes. But it was the right time to leave practice with the new emphasis on computers and an information explosion and my decreasing energy.

I think about my patients often and I confess, despite what I just said, I periodically call some of them to see how they are doing. I realize that it is really more for me than for them, but I try not to make that obvious. The hardest calls are when things aren't going that well and my caring is no longer as important as it was.

Bob and his family were patients of mine almost from the day I started. I attended their daughters' weddings, shared in their tragedies, cared for multiple illnesses, and counseled the children. When Bob was diagnosed with Alzheimer's, I told him it was very early and we would go through it together and learn from each other. Then I retired. He has gone on with good care but without me. I feel guilty.

I realize some of this is ego, a loss of importance, but mainly it is not fulfilling that promise and cheating myself out of the pleasure of learning and giving.

I was particularly close with Marylou and her family. I attended her mother's birthday parties, cared for her and her husband's chronic illnesses and undiagnosed illnesses, supported them through the illness and death of their daughter, and listened when that's all I could do. Last year she called me when she was diagnosed with breast cancer. I stayed in touch and expressed my pleasure when she did well. But I wasn't involved in the therapy decisions, wasn't there when it was time to cry or talk to the family. I feel incomplete.

There is a power that comes from being a doctor that can be dangerous, but when used for the benefit of the patient, that power can overwhelm many adversities. It is being their doctor that gives you that power.

Robin was diagnosed with prostate cancer about ten years ago. I saw him frequently for migraine headaches. He is a very bright guy who knows much about medicine and was always involved in his own decisions. When he was diagnosed he reminded me that we had discussed screening and he had chosen not to pursue it, even while I questioned myself. The follow-up letters from various urologists were not so understanding as they expressed a different opinion about screening. Recently I got a letter from a new urologist who obviously didn't know I was retired for over four years (or Robin didn't bother to tell her that he had a new doctor). I called Robin to see how he was after I forwarded the letter to his new doctor. As we talked Robin revealed that he had multiple complications requiring permanent catheters and had to give up work. I still felt some responsibility as he told me "I wish you were still in practice. I miss our talks." I feel humbled.

We spend so much time as doctors worrying about doing the right thing and giving the right advice that we sometimes forget that we need to have confidence in our patients and their ability to make their own decisions and accept the responsibility that goes along with that.

Jane called to get some advice with a problem they were having with her stepson. I listened, gave some suggestions about who to see, and offered to stay in touch. I had known Jane for years—rarely for herself as we together cared for her father, sister, and mother through their illnesses and death. She was still a caretaker and said she didn't know who else to call. I feel that it's hard to "be there" when you are not there.

In Loxtercamp's writing about "being there," he emphasizes that he doesn't mean always being there 24/7, but rather creating a state of mind for the patient that you will be there when they need you. I once talked with a patient of mine about the doctor-patient relationship in front of a class of first-year medical students. I asked her what was most important about our relationship. She said when she was diagnosed with diabetes, I gave her my private home phone number.

I responded, "Mrs. E, in our fifteen years together, how many times have you used that number?"

"None," was her immediate reply.

I really don't know if my retirement and our separation have been easier for my patients than for me. I certainly hope so. Part of my job was to encourage their independence and self-sufficiency. My emotional dependence on them is my problem and I suspect not that uncommon among doctors. I am still teaching and doing some research as some of my retired friends still go to grand rounds and travel to medical meetings even though they don't see any patients.

I have few regrets in retiring from my practice. I am happy and busy, but not in the same way as seeing patients. It was the right thing to do at the right time, and although I miss it every day, I feel so lucky to have been there for those previous forty-two years. I wish more young medical students understood this. Then there would be more students choosing family medicine careers and enjoying this most rewarding life.

Notes

1. Michael Balint, *The Doctor, His Patient, and the Illness* (London: Pitman Medical, 1957)
2. David Loxtercamp, "Being There: On the Place of the Family Physician," *Journal of the American Board of Family Practice* 4, no. 5 (1991): 354–60.

Part 2
Jonathan Han, MD

I have been a family physician for twenty-four years, during which time I have worked with the medically underserved and have taught family practice residents and medical students in San Francisco, Boston, and Pittsburgh. I am past the "middle" of my career, a milestone that I have difficulty acknowledging—not only because of concerns I have with aging, but also because I have never been one to scrupulously plan the years that lie ahead. Nevertheless, I've been blessed and am so grateful for the many opportunities that have presented themselves to me in a lifetime of work in family medicine.

Since childhood and on numerous occasions, from medical school admission essays to interviews with residents, I have said that I wanted to be a family physician. The first doctor I can remember was kindly Dr. Axthelm, whose sterile, spartan office was decorated with diplomas and Snellen eye charts on institutional green walls, featured impressive glass jars filled with cotton balls and tongue depressors on the shelves, and was always suffused with the smell of rubbing alcohol circulated by a creaky ceiling fan. And it had those silver metal syringes, which were huge back then—and I'm sure it's not just my childhood imagination playing tricks on me.

So my earliest conception of doctorhood was the affable family practitioner. The family doctors I knew saw patients out of venerable old brownstones, sat with the locals at the lunch counter of the village diner, and served on committees at City Hall. This community-involved life was part of family medicine.

I'm a second-generation Korean-American and my father was the first Korean protestant minister in Ohio, so growing up in predominantly white small-town Ohio in the late 1960s was in many ways an isolating experience. I didn't have any Asian (much less Korean) peers in school, and I had little exposure to Korean culture outside our home. Today there are hundreds of Korean churches in Ohio, a testament to the growth of the Korean-American community that was accelerated by the Immigration Act of 1965. Many Korean physicians, including surgeons and other specialists, came to the United States in the years following the Immigration Act and found work as general practitioners— "family doctors" in the small towns across the country.

That history of immigration and resettlement, of forging new identities and finding one's place in the world, has been of enormous interest to me, and I've tried to write about it in order to understand and also fully appreciate the challenges and blessings I live today. Family medicine has also evolved during these past forty years, becoming a board-certified, residency-trained specialty of its own. It has grown and changed over time while remaining true to its roots in "general practice" as embodied in the Norman Rockwell paintings of the friendly country doctor and the television persona of the kindly Marcus Welby, MD.

Storytelling is one of the most powerful ways we connect with each other, and I've always enjoyed it in its varied colorful forms. My mother enthralled me with stories of tranquil mountain hikes, dramatic athletic accomplishments, and harrowing escapes from Communists during the Korean War. My father told similar stories of the hardship and sacrifice, scholarship and generosity that strengthened his faith and resolve. From my parents, I learned to appreciate the twists and turns of conflict that characterized a good story, and I found that listening to people tell their stories helped me to understand myself.

That is why I chose family medicine as a career—even the name "family" medicine implies a specialty that values something bigger and more profound than any organ system or even the individual who is the sum of his or her anatomical parts. Family medicine values the whole story: the person, his or her relationships—failed, strained, and successful—and his or her place in the world. These are the stories I like to read, think about, and try to write about.

The following quotation from E.M. Forster expresses so well why I chose family medicine as a career and why I want to continue learning to write:

> *Only connect! That was the whole of her sermon.*
> *Only connect the prose and the passion, and both*
> * will be exalted,*
> *And human love will be seen at its height.*
> *Live in fragments no longer.*
> *Only connect...*
>
> —E.M. Forster, *Howards End*

The essays and poems that follow are included in chronological order. I was inspired to write the first two stories after attending a seminar on narrative medicine led by Paul Gross, who has guided many aspiring writers along the way. Writing about difficult patient care experiences helped me to find meaning in mistakes and to promise myself to do better the next time for my patients and myself.

Over the years, I found writing to be a necessary outlet to express frustration and disappointment in a fractured, inequitable health care system that should aspire to do more and often contentedly settles for much less. Drawing upon experiences from my training in San Francisco at the height of the AIDS epidemic, I wanted to channel my anger and frustration into the activism of the written word, following the examples of so many AIDS advocates who helped transform the care of the marginalized into a model of care that values every human being. It became my hope to motivate others to feel something, anything, when surveying the suffering and injustice that still exists within the broken landscape of our health care system.

Now I realize that if a reader feels something, anything, when engaging with my writing, it is reward enough—because it is that connection that is most important. And I find that the most satisfying aspect of my daily work as a family physician is in the relationships with patients, families, colleagues, students, residents, and mentors—all of which evolve and deepen with time and experience. Although health systems and professional organizations increasingly judge our efforts on the basis of "outcomes," it is these fundamentally complex and interesting human relationships that ultimately sustain us. And I find storytelling as important today as ever, as we move forward to reform health care—to preserve the value of connectedness.

One of my favorite quotes from Thomas Merton expresses this well:

Do not depend on the hope of results. You may have to face the fact that your work will be apparently worthless and even achieve no result at all, if not perhaps results opposite to what you expect. As you get used to this idea, you start more and more to concentrate not on the results, but on the value, the rightness, the truth of the work itself. You gradually struggle less and less for an idea and more and more for specific people. In the end, it is the reality of personal relationship that saves everything.

The Kindest Insult

That Mrs. Park wore a woolen overcoat and scarf on an unusually warm spring afternoon was not disconcerting to me. After all, this uniform is typical of many mentally ill elderly folk living a tenuous existence on the streets of San Francisco. Her paranoid rants about the end of the world and the neighbors who were spying on her also left me unmoved. What was painfully upsetting to me, however, was the anger and offence she took at my need for a Korean language interpreter.

Mrs. Park stopped growling and gesticulating long enough to appear hurt.

"If he is Korean, why does he need someone to speak his language for him?" Mrs. Park exhorted through the translator as she eyed me suspiciously. The interpreter shifted nervously through her own embarrassment as she channeled this message to me.

Having grown up in the only Korean family within several counties in rural Ohio, I did not place learning my "native tongue" high among my childhood priorities. Not that my immigrant parents didn't try to teach my brother and me the Korean language; but what language skills I did develop eventually withered away from lack of use and interest. After all, most of my peers were white, and learning the latest rules and nuances of popular culture were increasingly important as I grew older.

A fierce nationalism characterizes most Koreans, within which the primacy of identity is closely tied to fluency in the Korean language. During my first trip to Korea, taken after graduation from medical school, I vividly recall anger and embarrassment when a taxicab driver took a maliciously circuitous route around Seoul, in order that he could have more time to berate both my mother for not teaching me Korean and me for not being dutiful or interested enough to learn the language myself.

Koreans here and abroad have had an ambivalent relationship with the United States, stemming from many reasons—not least of which are the Korean War and the persistent division of North from South Korea, determined by forces from without the Korean Peninsula. The history of Korea is filled with episodic occupation by other countries, including Japan. Subsequently, the survival of Korean language and culture is testament to the nationalism, pride, and resistance to assimilation demonstrated by these "Irish of the East" through the centuries.

Now, as Mrs. Park interrogated me further about my psychological shortcomings related to my Korean muteness, I tried in vain to turn the tables on her and raise my own agenda.

"Please tell Mrs. Park that her blood test for syphilis is positive, and because of our concern for her mental illness, we would like to do a procedure called a spinal tap."

As the translator and I attempted to convey this message, Mrs. Park stopped growling and gesticulating long enough to appear hurt, instead of angry.

For a moment I imagined she was recollecting painful memories of a past life in Japan, where she served as a "comfort woman" for Japanese infantrymen during the Second World War. Stigmatized forever—reviled by both the Japanese, who had physically and sexually abused her; and the Koreans, who had spiritually disowned her—she became a woman with a language and culture but without a country.

This reflection was short lived, however, as she quickly resumed her diatribe of anger and insults, of which I made out a few threads, including "traitor" and "ingrate."

Frustrated at my inability to get on with a busy clinic schedule, I muttered in exasperation, "*Gijebeh.*" As a child, I had heard my mother and her friends use this word to describe any woman with whom they were angry or disappointed.

At this utterance, which translates roughly as "little girl," Mrs. Park's face lit up, and she laughed heartily, embracing my hands warmly. The translator even covered her mouth and giggled as she looked away from my confused gaze.

The act of calling an elderly woman a little girl within the Korean culture of hierarchy and filial piety should have been one of both great insult and disrespect. However, Mrs. Park stopped laughing long enough to shake my hand again, and to tell me that she would consent to the lumbar puncture. In fact, she genuinely connected with me after that visit, greeting me with a smile and often regaling me with stories of her youth during her subsequent office appointments.

I never asked her why she suddenly accepted my cultural naïveté or what motivated her to tolerate my inadvertent affront to Korean pride that was inherent in my inability to be a "native speaker." Perhaps my remark was the kindest insult she had ever received, which had arisen out of my desperation as a fellow Korean who, like her, was in many ways still a foreigner in America.

Welcome to the Arctic Circle

"You're a f—ing Korean!"

This was the greeting I received from a previously comatose twenty-five-year-old Eskimo woman, rudely awakened into a place of Narcan-induced hyperawareness and harsh ER examination room lights, as she suspiciously surveyed my face. Mine was the same face she had seen just three days before, as I repaired a laceration on her arm. On that visit, however, there was no such recognition, only a sigh of learned resignation.

The paramedics who accompanied her, two Inuit men who knew her well—who were familiar with her sad history of alcoholism, drug abuse and domestic violence—squirmed with embarrassment and barely concealed laughter.

"Welcome to the Arctic Circle," I thought to myself.

For a moment, I suspended my own disbelief as this somewhat comical but unfortunately all-too-familiar situation played out before me. I am a second-generation Korean American and was raised as one of the few Asian Americans in a mostly white, middle class, rural Ohio town. My father was the first Korean Protestant minister in Ohio, and he and my mother had quietly and bravely emigrated from Korea to Ohio some 45 years ago.

I grew up experiencing much racism and prejudice. Facing provocative racist taunts by children and adults alike and being ridiculed for my Asian features were painful reminders of my "perpetual foreigner" status. As a child, I was constantly encouraged by my parents to respond to racism by "ignoring other people's ignorance." This was reinforced by the silence of society at large—the topic of racism against Asians had not yet entered the public consciousness or debate. Like many children, I struggled with desires to conform, to be accepted by my non-Korean peers. Participating in athletics, including basketball, was one way I tried to "fit in." However, even as a collegiate varsity basketball player, I could not escape racist jeers by spectators at many of our games. Chants like "put the Chinaman in the game" were intimidating to me, and the sad irony that even athletic achievement could not spare me from ridicule was blatantly obvious.

Feeling somewhat lost, somewhere in between cultures of Korea and America, I searched for a place to fit in, to be anonymous, to not stand out simply because of my physical appearance. These struggles of identity intensified as I grew older, even as I moved toward a career in medicine.

One of the reasons I had chosen medicine in general and family medicine in particular was to be of service to others—to walk in my father's footsteps, as it were. I was drawn to working with the medically underserved, with those who had faced extra battles and who had suffered after missed or unavailable opportunities. Having worked in several Indian Health Service facilities, I had enjoyed the fact that my physical appearance resembled those of the Native Americans I served. After all, we were distant relatives, sharing ancestors who had crossed the Bering Straits land bridge. I enjoyed it when patients would ask, "What tribe are you from? Did you know my uncle?"

And yet here in the rural Arctic was a cruel reminder that it is human nature to first recognize the differences between each other before we affirm our similarities. I had forgotten how—within this tiny northern Alaskan village of 1,000 people, composed mostly of Eskimos—a small community of about fifty Koreans lived and thrived. These relative newcomers owned and operated four out of the five businesses in this Inuit town. Not far beneath the human tundra, however, there existed deep resentments between the Alaskan natives, who struggled with poverty and subsistence, and the Koreans, who were viewed as holding the purse strings. These conflicts were similar to those among Korean business owners and their predominantly African American neighbors and patrons in economically depressed areas of Los Angeles and Manhattan. Once again, the bitter determinants of "us" versus "them," though decided along racial lines, were rooted in both real and perceived disparities in wealth, power, and opportunity. Here in the frozen north among the Inuit, with whom I had naively felt a bond solely because of physical appearance and distant ancestry, I could not avoid the painful stereotyping and assumptions that arise when we separate ourselves from others by race and class.

As these thoughts flew in a flurry, or not, I suddenly turned to my hyperawake patient, who was now smiling with boldness and acuity, and replied, "In all my years of living in America, I've been called a chink, a jap, and a slant-eyed gook. This is the first time anyone ever correctly called me a Korean!"

She smiled even more broadly, and the Inuit paramedics now felt comfortable laughing out loud.

I added, "Now, you'll have to hold still while I insert this rubber tube into your nose to pump your stomach out."

Although I was the one now smiling broadly, the initial satisfaction I felt in the irony of the situation unfolding in this way was short-lived, giving way quickly to concerns about the seriousness of her medical condition.

If only my conflicting emotions of anger, vindication, and guilt were so short-lived.

Malignant Neglect

What brought Mrs. Waite (not her real name) to our emer-
gency department was the intervention of her husband of eleven
years. Frail, cachectic, unable to walk, Mrs. Waite glanced lovingly
at her husband from her hospital bed and said, "I didn't want to
come here." In a low, husky voice she continued, "He picked me
up and drove me here, against my wishes." Apparently, she deemed
the thirty-pound weight loss, sustained over the past two years,
relatively inconsequential. The longstanding vaginal discharge, the
odor of which was still redolent from the nurses' station down the
hall, had become for her a tolerable inconvenience. None of these
signs of a significant medical problem were cause for Mrs. Waite
to seek our help. Fortunately, her husband had finally experienced
enough and brought her to our emergency department.

As the teaching attending for a family practice inpatient
service, I was hoping to lead a knowledgeable discussion about
Mrs. Waite's illness. Her clinical presentation sounded relatively
straightforward moments before, as the senior resident described
her in rounds. "The patient is a thirty-eight-year-old, nulliparous
white woman with a medical history significant for congenital
adrenal hyperplasia (CAH), untreated twenty years, who is now
admitted with urinary tract infection, renal failure, and pelvic
pain." We reviewed her physical findings and laboratory studies.
We talked about her clinical manifestations of CAH, including
virilization, amenorrhea, and stress-induced adrenal insufficiency.
Why did her adrenal disease go untreated for so long? "Lack
of medical insurance," replied the resident without missing a
beat. As we discussed the causes of her renal failure, the resident

conjured up the CT scans of Mrs. Waite's abdomen and pelvis from the electronic medical record.

"There is a foreign body, stuck within a large calcified mass in her pelvis," observed the resident. Whatever it was, encased in a calcified cocoon of flesh within the vagina, it had grown so large that it occupied most of the pelvis and subsequently caused postobstructive renal failure.

At her bedside, the resident and I sat down to take a detailed history. Barely a skeletal 100 pounds, struggling to hold up her head, Mrs. Waite demonstrated remarkable candor and poise as she provided us with a road map of tragedy, lost and missed opportunities that led to this hospitalization. As we listened, I became preoccupied with the reasons why she neglected herself. What prevented her from receiving the care she so desperately needed?

The sentinel event most responsible for her predicament was a rape that occurred twelve years ago, shortly before she married her husband. She had gone to a party with some friends and had gotten drunk. She woke up the following morning naked, alone in a stranger's bed, with blood-stained sheets. She could not remember who raped her. She recalled a great deal of physical and emotional pain after the event, but like most women who have been sexually assaulted, she felt too ashamed and embarrassed to report the rape to the police or to seek legal help. Convinced that her complaint would not be taken seriously, she believed that being intoxicated made the assault her responsibility.

After the rape, she began to experience pelvic pain and malodorous vaginal discharge that would progressively worsen and become an ignominiously tolerable part of her life. Mrs. Waite was unable to have vaginal intercourse with her husband for the past 6 years because of dyspareunia and postcoital bleeding. However, she refused to seek medical attention initially because of her shame and guilt—and later, because she could not afford a gynecologic examination. When we informed her that a foreign body was present within the pelvic mass, Mrs. Waite immediately identified it as an object used in the assault. "He must have put that in me when he raped me," she concluded, shaking her head. Her calm acceptance of this news represented a sad justification for the years of anger and blame she had directed toward herself. She felt, perversely, that she "deserve[d] to have this thing" as a horrible reminder of the assault.

Mrs. Waite was depressed for years after the rape. Her obsessive feelings of remorse and regret continued to haunt her. The spectrum of signs she exhibited, including social isolation and alcohol abuse, were indicative of posttraumatic stress disorder (PTSD). She never became suicidal, and her self-neglect was not an overt sign of intentional self-injury. She never sought help from the rape crisis center nor the community mental health professional, telling us the stigma of seeing a psychotherapist and her inability to afford counseling without insurance prevented her from doing so. Over the past twelve years, without the benefit of formal therapy, she gradually "felt better" and was not depressed at the time of her hospitalization.

Alcoholism also impaired Mrs. Waite's judgment significantly. She had had problems with alcohol abuse as a teenager, but the rape precipitated a downward spiral toward alcoholism in the years to follow. She began drinking a bottle of Black Velvet every couple of days "because it helped my pain." Fortunately, her alcoholism remitted in the past year, though her newfound sobriety was achieved at the cost of her increasing incapacity.

Whether Mr. Waite enabled his wife's self-neglect was unclear: How could he passively accept her progressive physical decline and alcoholism? By her account, however, Mr. Waite's emotional support never wavered during the past eleven years. Indeed, the spiritual sustenance he provided was probably the key factor in "treating" her depression over the years.

The final obstacles that prevented Mrs. Waite from getting medical care were her lack of health insurance and the scarcity of clinicians for the uninsured. The Waites lived in a town located within a federally designated medically underserved area. Only one sporadically staffed "free clinic" and one family-planning clinic were available to provide care to uninsured patients, and the Waites were unaware of these resources. To make matters worse, even if Mrs. Waite had qualified for Medicaid, many local clinicians did not accept Medicaid patients because of low reimbursement, so outpatient health care would have been just as inaccessible to her.

Although the United States has a predominantly employer- or work-based health insurance system, many businesses do not offer health insurance to their employees as a cost-saving measure. Mrs. Waite lost her medical insurance after high school, despite working for various small businesses over the years. Without insurance, she could not afford to see her endocrinologist, and she stopped her steroid therapy twenty years ago. Her husband, a self-employed truck driver, was also uninsured. Paying for his truck and keeping it running took priority over health insurance. The Waites did not seek medical care except for emergencies. The concepts of "health care maintenance" and "primary care provider" were utterly foreign to them, as they would be to millions of their uninsured and underinsured peers.

As her story unfolded, it was apparent that Mrs. Waite had sailed into the perfect storm of terrible circumstances: her unevaluated and untreated rape, resulting in depression, PTSD, and alcoholism; her lack of health insurance; and the paucity of local resources to provide health care for the uninsured. Her pathological decision not to seek help was enabled by a prevailing culture that stigmatizes survivors of rape and those with mental illness or substance abuse. Punctuating her sentences with an unsettling, emaciated smile, Mrs. Waite continued in a calm baritone: "I'm not afraid of dying. But I want to get better and support my husband like he supported me."

Four days in the hospital had gone by, at a cost exceeding $29,000. The urosepsis and renal failure resolved with bilateral nephrostomies, antibiotics, corticosteroids, and hydration. The consultants agreed that surgery to remove the pelvic mass could be temporarily deferred, until Medicaid coverage could be obtained. Mrs. Waite was discharged home; the etiology of the pelvic mass remaining a mystery.

Together we completed reams of paperwork as she applied for Medicaid, which was denied because Mr. Waite had $2,000 of assets in excess of eligibility guidelines. We discussed the growing possibility that the Waites were heading toward bankruptcy, since medical catastrophe is the primary cause of financial loss for more than half of debtors filing for bankruptcy.[1] Meeting Medicaid eligibility guidelines after going broke would be no silver lining for the Waites.

An exploratory laparotomy was finally performed four months later, after Mrs. Waite's parents loaned her money to defray some of the expenses. When the 771-gram, $15 \times 8 \times 5$–centimeter oblong petrified mass was removed, it was sawed apart in the operating room, revealing a 4.5×3.5–centimeter black plastic vessel that appeared to be a shot glass. Surrounded by concentric layers of calcified tissue, the shot glass had taken on a life of its own and had nearly taken the life of its "owner."

The surgery proceeded without complication, and her postoperative course was uneventful. She was sent home six days later, at a cost exceeding $30,000. Facing further reconstructive surgery and struggling to make payments on her hospitalizations, Mrs. Waite remains sober and confident. "I'm a people person, I'll be all right," she explained optimistically. What about that shot glass? Mrs. Waite responded with stoic acceptance, "I don't know what that sick bastard was thinking when he put that in me. But it's over now, and I have to move on."

Move on, indeed. The final identification of a shot glass, expanding within her flesh and threatening her life as would any malignancy, seemed anticlimactic. The twelve years of pain and anguish accrued along the way represent a tragedy made worse by the many ways her suffering could have been alleviated. A dozen years ago, a simple pelvic examination—with removal of the foreign body as well as screening and treatment for depression, PTSD, and alcohol abuse—could have prevented this cascade of events. Unfortunately, many barriers to health care, acting together in complex concert, made that relatively low-tech solution impossible. We will never know if she could have ameliorated her pain by seeking care earlier had she been insured, as she claims she would have.

At first glance, I was sadly struck by Mrs. Waite's self-neglect; undoubtedly, her alcoholism and depression impaired her judgment and prevented her from seeking medical care in the first weeks and months after the rape. I soon realized, however, that the responsibility for this malignant neglect is shared by society and by our medical community. Perhaps the greatest tragedy is that, as years passed and her medical complications progressed, Mrs. Waite believed her health problems were not worth profession-al attention until death was imminent. Her fear of the financial cost of receiving care convinced her to prioritize her health below other matters of less ultimate importance. This dehumanizing indoctrination, whereby patients—as well as medical profession-als—buy into the concept of health care as a commodity and not an essential human right, is the most perverse outcome of a system that is readily available only to those fortunate enough to have "qualified" for insurance. Mrs. Waite's story is a painful reminder of the suffering that goes on largely unnoticed in our communities every day. Our hope, as medical professionals, is that we find new ways of working collaboratively to provide comprehensive health care to all people, regardless of ability to pay. Our challenge is to prevent another terribly unfortunate case of malignant neglect in the future.

Acknowledgment

I would like to thank Royal Rhodes, PhD, Marilyn Fitzgerald, PhD, and Kevin Grumbach, MD, for their editorial assistance.

Note: The patient described in this essay read the manuscript and gave written permission to publish her story.

Notes

1. David U. Himmelstein, Elizabeth Warren, Deborah Thorne, and Steffie Woolhandler, "MarketWatch: Illness and Injury as Contributors to Bankruptcy," *Health Affairs* (February 2005), published exclusively online at http://content.healthaffairs.org/content/suppl/2005/01/28/hlthaff.w5.63.DC1/

Procedure Note

Finish the note.

Because I was so relieved that my patient was still alive, I almost forgot to document in his medical record the events that had just unfolded.

"Patient is an eighteen-year-old Eskimo male with self-inflicted gunshot wound to the right chest."

We were somewhere above the Arctic Circle, 400 miles from the nearest surgeon, and I had to act. Having just transported him by seaplane to our outpost hospital, I was filled with adrenaline-laced expectations that I could help him. Although our tiny eight-bed hospital resembled a sessile MASH unit more than the sprawling county hospital where I had trained, our medical staff was quite familiar with handling traumatic injuries, as life above permafrost was rife with adventure and misfortune. "The Arctic is unforgiving," the charge nurse dryly observed as she greeted us at the door.

As a family physician, I had limited experience performing operative procedures, and my young patient required one that I had never done before. It was early in my career, and I was not afraid to attempt something risky and new. Buoyed by romantic notions of practicing in the Alaskan "bush" country, I relished the role of playing the lone country doc, relying on my guts as well as wits to meet the needs of my patients. Harming anyone through my own inexperience, I selfishly rationalized, was one of the unavoidable risks local folks assumed in living an isolated arctic existence.

I took a deep breath and quickly reviewed a surgical text-book that made the task appear straightforward enough; surely the tidy description of events would fall into place after the obligatory sterile prep. Bearing down, harder and harder, I suddenly pierced his chest cavity with the trocar.

All at once, his fascia and pleura, blood and breath gave way with terrible finality—like thin ice collapsing under the weight of an unsupervised child. His bright red blood, along with my barely concealed hubris, gushed from this new chest wound, filling me with a nauseating fear that I had mistakenly pierced a major artery and killed my patient.

"Everything will be all right," I told my patient, and myself, as I busily connected drains, checked intravenous lines and cardiac monitors, feigning calmness as I palpated my own thready pulse. Slowly, over thirty minutes, my suppressed panic subsided as his hemorrhaging slowed to a trickle. The most reassuring sign that my patient would survive was that the trademark unflappability of the grizzled charge nurse returned, replacing the uncharacteristic wide-eyed worry she wore just moments before. I had been granted a temporary reprieve.

Finish the note, I reminded myself. Opening my patient's medical chart, I scribbled a few mechanical phrases, designed to satisfy my partners and nursing staff, as well as the potential readership of malpractice attorneys. I described in bland detail the indications for the procedure; the obtaining of necessary consents; and an account of incisions made, scalpels used, and sutures closed. Ending my note, "Patient tolerated emergency thoracostomy without complication," I signed my name with an undeservedly confident flourish. I should have been humbled by the irony that my note implied comfortable routine instead of the bloody fear I had experienced just moments before. Instead, I reveled in my survivorship, nurturing the hubris that had propelled me into that life-threatening situation in the first place and deferring lessons about humility to the long night ahead.

Writing with a newly steady hand, telling my side of the story using professionally sparse language, served as another initiation rite into the medical fraternity of "those who see this all the time." Ritually following the script of the revered SOAP note—an appropriate acronym for the patient's *Subjective* complaints, *Objective* findings, *Assessment* by physician, and *Plan* of action—I imposed a cleanliness and orderliness on the emotionally soiled and chaotic events that characterize medical encounters. I did not mention any of the distinctly human but clinically less expedient facts, such as the details of my patient's strained family relationships, poverty, and nearly fatal sense of isolation and despair. As we lifted him from stretcher to seaplane just an hour ago, he surveyed the crowd of curious villagers who had gathered at the spectacle—and observed without irony, "I didn't know so many people cared."

But my procedure note was not the place for this reflection, nor for any admission of my own insecurity and vulnerability to error. I had been trained to translate first-person accounts of illness into secondhand reporting, filtering away details and creating an altogether new though not unbiased story following the directive: If it's not in the note, it didn't happen. Every medical role model marching ahead of me—attending, resident, or senior medical student—documented his or her work in the same terse, emotionally vacant hand. Although every procedure note I wrote was purportedly about my patient, I was ultimately saying something about me, about the kind of doctor I wanted to be: organized in approach, thorough in thought, and—above all—correct in judgment. Hundreds of notes a week would be written in this fashion, fragments and roadmaps of patient encounters that define a profession and mark change and growth. As long as the patient outcome was good, or at worst unavoidably bad through no fault of my own, I did not feel compelled to reconcile the differences between the story I wrote and the story my patient and I actually shared. But the discord between the acceptably documented and the movingly undocumented remained, reminding me the way a phantom limb pain does that the integrity of connection was missing and needed to be addressed.

Returning to my patient's bedside, I was met by a stout Inuit babushka wearing the ubiquitous mirror sunglasses and puffy, fur-lined parka essential to life in the Arctic. After she introduced herself as the teen's aunt, we had a conversation that rivaled my written note in brevity. In the face of the stoic demeanor of many Eskimos, I described the recent events in an unintentionally culturally congruent manner. Barely disclosing the untold hazards that lay ahead or the dangers that he had already faced in my inexperienced hands, I cautioned coolly, "He's not out of the woods yet." Nodding thoughtfully, she thanked me and quietly padded out of the room. It didn't occur to me that trees and forests were a long way from the endless barren tundra where we lived.

I documented this brief conversation in his chart: "Family member aware of seriousness of his condition." This cursory statement left the impression that we had communicated on some significant level. However, the unspoken feelings and omitted details would have told a more compelling story. Sometimes the constraints we impose on ourselves as physicians are revealed not only in these efficiently shallow notes but also in the problems we dare to address and act upon.

I briefly recalled the exhilaration I felt knowing my suicidal patient would survive my first thoracostomy, and now I was grateful for the opportunity to face the challenging problem of his depression. However, my confidence wielding scalpels or antibiotics contrasted with the inadequacy I felt taking care of seemingly more intractable problems like mental illness, domestic violence, and substance abuse. Despite my best efforts to provide support, psychiatric referrals, and medications, would he continue to abuse drugs or his partner and drift toward worsening depression and a repeat of attempted suicide?

Patience and perseverance, not surgical dexterity, were now required—skills that he and I would need to develop together on the path to recovery.

My pager interrupted this reverie, and I moved on through the night shift, putting out smaller medical fires along the way. It was a blessing to keep busy, to not dwell on doubts and regrets that would slow me down. Folks with sore throats, community-acquired pneumonias, and other problems I had seen hundreds of times before were seen and treated with ease. All that was really needed for most of these patients was reassurance, limit setting, and a tincture of time. That surly, recently divorced fellow pacing gingerly in Room 2, I described as the "Grade I ankle sprain." My medical shorthand focused attention on the acute problem, the patient's "complaint," instead of the complete person. What salvaged my note to convey a deeper human connection was the closing phrase, "follow-up visit in 2–3 weeks." The return appointment was my promise to continue this collaboration between neophyte professional and seasoned amateur, and to attend to his angry mood, as well as his injured ankle, next time.

Another piercing sequence of beeps, and I was on my way back to the emergency room, where I met a teenage male, sixteen years old, who sustained a "boxer's fracture" of the right hand during a fight with a gang member from a neighboring village.

Booming bass and tinny percussion blared from headphones slung across his neck as he sized me up and identified my Korean heritage solely by looking at my face. It was not just a good guess; he was familiar with a small cadre of Koreans who had immigrated to his village as business owners. These new settlers were resented by the native Alaskans who, in their relative poverty and subsistence existence, felt exploited. As I finished splinting his hand, we exchanged stories—he was curious about my experiences with racism. Enlightened despite the behavior of many of his townspeople, he thought it was wrong to discriminate against the local Koreans because of race or socioeconomic status. "Those Koreans are just trying to get by like the rest of us," he reassured me as he shared stories about bigotry among whites, Eskimos, and Koreans above the Arctic Circle.

For the first time all night, I felt relaxed as we talked about similar conflicts I faced growing up in the lower forty-eight. Here was an opportunity to build a relationship, utilizing skills with which I had more confidence than handling scalpels and trocars. This was an important "teaching moment" I could use to help him avoid another fight in the future.

Emboldened by the rapport I thought we shared in this moment, flush with confidence in having competently immobilized his fracture with an ulnar gutter splint, I reminded him that he had just broken his hand during a fight with another teen whose only transgression was membership in a rival gang. "He was just running with a different crowd. After all we just talked about, don't you think that was a bit hypocritical?"

His response to my verbal intervention was immediate. "Who are you calling a hypocrite, fool?" he spat at me. Shaking his newly-casted fist, he strode angrily out of the emergency room, our brief connection collapsed under the brute force of my ill-chosen words.

I had barely begun composing rationalizations, stewing in anger and regret, when a familiar Eskimo babushka trundled up to my side. She was as stoic as before, but her anger was unmistakable. "How dare you call my cousin a hypocrite," she seethed. "That isn't right."

This town was growing smaller by the minute.

"I'm sorry," I stammered, sincerely but with some smugness as I clung to my recent fortunes stabilizing fractures and evacuating chest wounds. She shook her head knowingly, glaring as she quietly left the room, recriminations echoing in the footfall of her mukluks.

Finish the damn note.

"Non-displaced fracture of the right fifth metacarpal, immobilized with ulnar gutter splint applied in the usual manner." There were many secrets edited out of this unsatisfying note, though the undisclosed story line this time was not about fear, inexperience, or—as always—uncertainty. Instead, my verbal heavy-handedness threatened to perpetuate or worsen existing fracture lines within a tiny Arctic community.

Had I slowed down enough to let my patient reflect on his own about his actions, both he and I could have learned a more powerful lesson. Instead, I was now faced with the painful challenge of repairing this latest iatrogenic complication, caused by my misuse of words sharper than any trocar.

Although it felt disingenuous to end the procedure note describing only the medically expedient issue of the boxer's fracture, I did not know how to document my error. No trusty textbook protocol for "mistake management" was available for consultation. Important questions remained, immediately selfish: How can I save face in the presence of my peers and community? Only later did the most meaningful question arise: How do I treat my patient as I would want to be treated, within a relationship complete with honesty, integrity, and all the risks of failure and disappointment?

Finish the note.

"We discussed and disagreed upon issues related to his injury."

My procedure note betrayed a clinical detachment I desired—as if I were the disciplined physician who had unerringly exercised the correct diagnostic and therapeutic techniques, with good outcomes, for years on end. However, I was not that coldly competent clinician depicted in my writing—instead, I was a struggling participant, wrestling again with regret, whose concern for this patient lay not with mending broken bones but with a blown opportunity for healing.

An apology was in order. To be faithful to my text, I had to first be faithful to my patient. This reconciliation required a combination of humble intention and luck, and I could do something about the first contingency only. I carefully printed my name, legibly, and closed his chart.

My shift had come to an end. After unceremoniously signing outpatient care responsibilities to my caffeinated partner, I slid on my parka and headed out of the hospital into the midnight sun of an Arctic summer. As I shuffled my way home, I spotted a familiar young man with a fresh cast on his arm, straddling one of those ubiquitous balloon-tired all-terrain vehicles. Our eyes met briefly, and when he didn't curse me or drive away in a cloud of dust, I interpreted his staying as yet another potential "teaching moment," this time for me.

"Wait up," I called as I walked toward him, hoping to set our broken relationship right in person, and to write a healthier ending to his story.

Acknowledgment

The author would like to thank Royal Rhodes, PhD, Marilyn Fitzgerald, PhD, and Audrey Young, MD, for their editorial comments and support.

Serious Side Effects

It was September 2007, and I hadn't seen Mr. Waite in more than a year. A few months before his last visit, I'd diagnosed him with prostate cancer, and he'd started radiation and hormone therapy, tolerating numerous side effects with stoic acceptance. Then his health insurance premiums rose to unaffordable heights—and three months into his cancer treatment, he'd lost his insurance coverage. Unable to afford care on his own, he'd stopped being treated.

From years of caring for patients like Mr. Waite, I've learned to compromise. Cobbling together treatment plans requires resourcefulness, accepting the uncertainties of undertreating versus not treating, and learning to respect patients who must give their health lower priority. I was as frustrated as Mr. Waite by the limited medical care and medications available to the uninsured and underinsured.

At the same time, in order for our society to provide sustained health care for all, we need effective cost control, and evidence-based prescribing practices are an essential part of achieving that. Many doctors don't use—and discourage the use of—free drug samples, because they contribute extraordinary costs to US health care. In 2005 alone, the pharmaceutical industry spent $18.4 billion on drug samples. Whether the costs of drug samples and the industry's other promotional activities (e.g., direct-to-consumer advertising) contribute directly to rising retail drug prices is a matter of debate; many doctors think there is, indeed, a direct relationship.

In response to these concerns, the Academic Medical Center for which I work drafted a Conflict of Interest (COI) policy restricting physician access to proprietary drug samples. Because we wanted to support our indigent patients yet abide by these COI directives, the Family Health Centers where I care for patients implemented "a hybrid drug distribution model," providing needy patients with medications that mix generic drugs and carefully selected brand-name drug samples. What we came up with is only a short-term solution; one that enables and incentivizes a profoundly broken health care system to remain unchanged. Ultimately, a safety net woven from a patchwork of work-arounds of this sort isn't financially or physically sustainable—and there already isn't enough time for the majority of physicians to support efforts like ours. Nor should they have to.

Unfortunately, our efforts could not reverse the course of events for Mr. Waite, whose prostate cancer had worsened during the months he was unable to afford his treatments. Despite the medications we provide through our hybrid drug program, he was once again beginning to sacrifice some expensive medications he still had to buy as his cancer progressed and his family's utility bills rose even higher. During a recent visit, Mr. Waite and I talked about his ongoing efforts—and frustrations—in trying to make ends meet. Would we be having this conversation, I wondered, if he'd been able to keep his health insurance and continue treatment for his prostate cancer? And would he now need all of these expensive new medications for his worsened problems, some of which aren't available either as samples or as generics?

In the health center where I work, we care for the "worried well" and the critically ill, the morbidly obese and the recalcitrant bulimic, the deeply depressed and the recovering alcoholic, the ex-con and the college provost. Taken as a whole, these patients represent every permutation of wealth and insurance status (including the complete lack of it). Compassionate, patient-centered medicine calls for physicians to respond empathically and care for every patient, validating each individual as unconditionally deserving of care. Is it possible for us to recapture the altruistic spirit expressed in our medical school admission essays and to embrace the idealism of Hippocrates and Maimonides, whose oaths and prayers we recite at medical school commencement ceremonies?

In the United States, we haven't yet addressed the fundamental question of whether health care is a human right, nor have we yet solved how to reverse disparities and improve quality of care for all patients. The way it works now, allocating limited medical resources is often determined by who is "deserving" versus who is "undeserving"—a malignant form of neglect.

In my opinion, Academic Medical Centers must take the lead in advocating not only for greater accountability in conflicts of interest but also for equal access to high-quality medical care for all. I believe that the example set by the academic community can, indeed, promote change. As Jerome Kassirer, former editor of the *New England Journal of Medicine*, wrote in 1995, "Market-driven health care creates conflicts that threaten medical professionalism." Millions of patients and health care professionals still worry about that.

Passing the Torch:
A Day in the Life of an
Attending Physician

Time fell back three days ago, leaving me one less hour of daylight to enjoy on a gorgeous Indian summer Wednesday. I'm the attending physician on a busy family medicine inpatient service, and it's been a long week of patient care and meetings. I rushed out of the hospital somewhere near 5:00 p.m., hoping to go for a short run before the season changes to winter.

Pulling out of the parking lot, the traffic slows to a crawl as both patients and pedestrians preoccupied with conversation meander through the crosswalk. I open my window to feel the warm fall breeze, reflecting on my day.

7:00 a.m.: I attended morning report led by our family medicine residents, briefly discussing patients in the hospital and their plans of action. Oatmeal and raisins, faux Egg McMuffin sandwiches, caffeine, and adrenaline fuel much of the conversation, which focuses on serious problems and crises in management, punctuated by frustrations dealing with care managers and insurance plan medical directors who constantly remind the residents that they need to discharge patients home as soon as possible.

In recent years, the Length of Stay (LOS) patients experience when hospitalized for medical and surgical care has decreased due to better treatments and concerted efforts to avoid nosocomial complications associated with prolonged hospitalization.

However, these shortened hospital stays have created new problems: patients are sent home with less resolution of their acute illness, forcing physicians and hospital staff to manage increased patient turnover and associated communication and cross-coverage issues. Have we reached a safety plateau where hospital LOS cannot be cut any shorter?

The residents wrap up their morning report rounds with a thank-you to the departing night coverage team and a plan to reconvene in a couple hours to further review patient care as a team.

7:30 a.m.: On to an administrative meeting, learning about imminent plans by Medicare to dramatically cut reimbursements to hospitals and physicians for patients readmitted to the hospital within thirty days for certain diagnoses, such as COPD (chronic obstructive pulmonary disease), CHF (congestive heart failure), asthma, and pneumonia. CMS (Center for Medicare and Medicaid Services) had introduced these regulations to cut costs under the guise of improving "quality" of care. Although there is no evidence that such a reimbursement strategy actually improves medical outcomes, we were warned that there will be widespread adoption of this non-reimbursement strategy. I told the group of a recent study in the VA hospital system that demonstrated no improvement in thirty-day readmissions despite the use of an integrated electronic information system and robust multidisciplinary discharge team follow up. Researchers had concluded that the reasons why patients with chronic illness were readmitted within thirty days were complicated and multifactorial, not simply the result of poor physician or hospital staff practice.[1]

Gnashing of teeth followed shortly thereafter.

The cars in front of me begin to move slowly, the earthy aromas of fall mixed with automobile exhaust, directing my attention to a group of three people standing at the corner ahead. As the traffic halts again, I recall a few conversations of the day.

10:30 a.m.: Our team spent the past four days taking care of a 53-year-old lady, Ms. M., suffering from schizophrenia, admitted to our hospital after a fall and syncopal episode. This was her third admission to a third different hospital within the past six weeks. She had undergone extensive cardiac and neurological testing during the previous two hospitalizations, yet she was discharged back to her personal care home (PCH) with no follow-up with a PCP (primary care physician) and had not been started on medications for her heart, cholesterol, and diabetes as advised during the two admissions. One hospital note from a previous admission stated, "No PCP located, so no one contacted." Ms. M. is well on her way toward joining the desperate statistic that the seriously mentally ill in our country die, on average, twenty-five years younger than their mentally "healthy" counterparts.

Despite the fact she could barely walk with her cane and walker, Ms. M. lives on the second floor of the PCH, which has no elevator. Ms. M. felt isolated to the second floor, frequently falling when she tried to negotiate the steps. During this hospital stay, Ms. M. worked with neurologists plus physical and occupational therapists to optimize her ambulation. Our team contacted a community mental health organization to confirm guardianship arrangements and to ensure that care management services would be in place. We also notified Adult Protective Services to help monitor her care while new housing arrangements could be made. The resident and medical student spent several hours making phone calls and networking with these agencies, even locating a PCP (Primary Care Practitioner) who would assume responsibility for her care upon discharge.

After all these efforts to care for Ms. M. and hopefully prevent another early readmission, we were informed later in the afternoon by her insurance company that the last two days of her four-day admission would be "denied" and not reimbursed. Time-consuming appeals processes would surely follow.

During our afternoon rounds, I reminded the team that today was the first day Ms. M. smiled. I told her I enjoyed her change in demeanor, and Ms. M. told me in a flat affect, without a trace of irony, "I like to smile."

The line of cars begins to move again. It's so warm, I may be able to wear shorts one last time this fall if I can make it to the park in time for my run.

12:30 p.m.: The medical student and I spent twenty minutes convincing Mr. G., a forty-two-year-old Cubs fan (obvious from the baseball hat constantly affixed to his head the previous three days), that he should not smoke cigarettes prior to surgery the following day. Mr. G. had been admitted with a partial bowel obstruction and was understandably restless. He told us he wanted to go for a walk outside to enjoy the sun, and really just wanted a smoke to unwind. After complaining about the bowel preparation for surgery, the too-soft mattress, and the incessant beeping noises that kept him awake the night before, he promised not to smoke if we would just let him go outside. We acquiesce.

I'm getting closer to the last stop sign before I leave the hospital campus and head home for my run. I guess there are thirty minutes of daylight left. As I approach the crosswalk, the three people standing on the corner are becoming familiar to me.

2:45 p.m.: The intern and I walk into the room to talk to Mr. B., a sixty-two-year-old man admitted for the fourth time in the past three weeks complaining of worsening abdominal pain due to chronic alcoholic pancreatitis. He was transferred to the medical floor from our emergency room, his thirty-sixth visit to his fourth hospital in the past nine weeks. As we enter the room, we are greeted by a shrouded figure moaning and lying motionless in a fetal position, a single scaly dry foot protruding from the bottom of the hospital bed.

"Mr. B.," we call to him. His head emerges from the sheet, graying temples framing an angry scowl and half-opened eyes.

"I want my pain meds," he announces.

The intern explains that we are not going to give him narcotic pain medications, that his laboratory tests are unremarkable, and that his radiologic findings are not too concerning.

"I want my pain meds, I told you," he repeats.

The intern and I sit down and talk to him for twenty-five minutes. We ask him about his past history of detox and rehab admissions, the revolving door of primary care physicians he has seen and not seen, and his willingness to receive treatment for his depression. Mr. B. tells us that he is not suicidal and names the various addiction specialists and AA (Alcoholics Anonymous) and NA (Narcotics Anonymous) meetings he has frequented in the past. Then Mr. B. asks if we are going to give him narcotics on this admission. We tell him we will not, that we would consult pain management specialists and work with him to address his pain and depression without narcotics.

Mr. B. rolls his eyes, pulls the sheet back over his head, and swears as we walk out of the room. Shortly afterward, Mr. B. signs himself out of the hospital AMA (Against Medical Advice).

I'm pumping the brakes, crawling to a rolling stop as I eye the three figures huddled in front of a bus shelter. One of our hospital security officers is sharing a laugh with Mr. G., sporting his Cubs hat and hospital gown. Mr G. is pointing toward something in the distance past the rows of stop lights, and he is smoking.

3:35 p.m.: An infectious-diseases specialist stops me in the hall to review a few of our complicated patients. In particular, Mr. K., a forty-three-year-old man who regularly uses cocaine, was being treated for a badly infected bite wound on his arm sustained while trying to "break up a fight between two dogs." Though we speculated why he was being attacked by dogs so frequently (this was his third dog bite in the past month), our team was worried about how he would care for his wound when he was discharged. We planned to send him home today and become his new PCP (Primary Care Practitioner) in order to provide close outpatient follow-up of his wounds, but the infectious diseases specialist wanted to keep him just a few more days in the hospital, suspecting that the patient would "bounce back" quickly with worsening infection if he left today.

After our team agreed to keep Mr. K. in the hospital, the infectious disease consultant told me with appropriate concern that he thought our residents sometimes discharge patients out of the hospital too quickly. We talk about the immense pressures the residents and attending staff face from care managers and insurance companies to discharge patients with less resolution of their acute illness, in an attempt to avoid denials of reimbursement. As a specialist, he admits that he doesn't have to deal with these daily conversations, defending and rationalizing the care we provide simply to avoid an insurance denial. We speculated with dread about the future of hospitals and our profession as reimbursement is squeezed, patient care acuity rises, and increasingly rapid turnover of patients escalates cross-coverage and communication problems.

A week later, I receive a letter from the insurance company telling me Mr. K's last three days of his six-day hospitalization—including intravenous antibiotics, wound care, and specialist follow-up—were "denied."

3:50 pm. I am meeting with our senior resident to review team management strategy when one of our pulmonary-specialist colleagues walks in the staff lounge looking for a bagel. We talk about the upcoming CMS denials of reimbursement for readmissions for certain chronic illnesses and conditions. Of these "preventable" problems, COPD, DVT (deep vein thrombosis), and c.diff (clostridium difficile) colitis are especially meaningful since the pulmonologist co-manages our intensive care unit. The bureaucrats who came up with this plan have forgotten this important fact: despite our following all the best evidence-based guidelines for DVT prophylaxis, handwashing, gowning, glov-

ing, alcohol-wiping our stethoscopes, and compulsive central line care, there will always be a few patients who get clots, line infections, and c.diff infections. MRSA (methicillin resistant staphylococcus aureus) and c.diff are already widespread in the community, and they will happen here. Despite our best efforts to provide our COPD patients with necessary medications, education, immunizations, and nutritional counseling, some patients will always smoke, get sick when the weather gets cold, and experience the unavoidable life stressors that get them in trouble with their breathing. We just don't have complete control over our patients and their lives. The bureaucrats that impose these regulations forget that shit happens.

I come to a complete stop at the crosswalk. Mr. G. smiles and taps an ash onto the sidewalk. I then realize the third man standing in the group is Mr. B. He is barely recognizable now as he stands there wearing rumpled slacks and a blue overstuffed sweater, throwing his head back laughing with Mr. G. and the security officer, slapping his thigh with one hand and holding a cigarette with his other. That salt-and-pepper hair and scraggly beard confirm his identity. I wonder what they are laughing at, but then again, I don't want to know.

4:20 p.m.: One of my family medicine faculty partners and I are talking about our grant-funded, evidence-based integrated behavioral and physical health care initiative, which will help our patients access the mental health services they need onsite in our primary care office. We are excited at the prospect of strengthening our Medical Home and improving the quality of life for our patients and their families, yet we worry that this model of care might not be financially sustainable because there are, at present, no consistently reliable plans to reimburse us for this care among our multiple third-party payors.

The "hotspotting" work done by Dr. Jeff Brenner of the Camden Health Coalition[2] in caring for the medically under-

served, especially those patients who are "high service utilizers," demonstrate that patient-centered care not only improves outcomes but dramatically decreases costs. Brenner identified the 1 percent of patients who account for over 30 percent of health care costs in his community, finding them localized in "hotspots" within public housing and other poverty-stricken locales. One particularly "hot" patient Brenner identified utilized more than $3.5 million of heath care services in five years. Brenner and his team of visiting nurses, social workers, and community health workers used creative outreach methods to provide care for these patients, preventing unnecessary ER (emergency room) visits and hospitalizations. In spite of this innovative work, Dr. Brenner has also met many obstacles in getting reimbursed by the third-party payers who are saving money from his work providing cost-effective, high-quality, patient-centered care.

My partner and I discuss the paradox of the public health perspective on Brenner's "hotspotting" work: throwing so many resources at the few most costly users goes against the directive of caring for the greatest number of patients with the limited resources that are available. Today, however, our efforts to "bend the cost curve" require not only creative solutions but new rationalizations of how we care for others and where our responsibilities for patient care begin and end. Mr. B. is clearly one of these "hot" patients racking up immense health care costs unchecked. Could Mr. B. benefit from more intense outreach? What team can facilitate change in his lack of insight, his lack of motivation for self-care? And what incentive does any primary care physician have to assume responsibility for his care? Mr. B. would certainly drag down any Pay For Performance (P4P) or quality measure score any physician would hope to attain to demonstrate her worthiness to payors or potential patients. And who would reimburse that doctor for the immense time and effort it would take to help Mr. B. change his behavior?

Today, I am only too happy to pass this torch to someone else. But who will take it from me?

I look at my watch. It's 5:03 p.m. I have just enough time to throw on my shorts and go for that run. Lying in my hammock is a worthy option also. I drive away from the hospital campus, leaving Mr. G. and Mr. B. behind, laughing and smoking in my rearview mirror.

We are not health care providers. We are, in fact, health care enablers—the healthy and worried well, motivated to optimize their health, come to us for advice and encouragement. The fortunate insured come to our offices and we enable them access to quality illness care, "health maintenance," and support. The uninsured, unmotivated, or unreachable behind societal and institutional barriers remain hidden and out of touch, meeting us transiently and expensively in crisis—in our hospitals because our present models of care delivery rely on patients to meet us where we are, not where they are. Within our broken system, we enable them to stay expensively out of sight. Health care policymakers and administrators continue to move the responsibility for increasing costs onto the physicians and hospitals themselves, implicitly placing the "blame" for illness and bad outcomes on physicians. Meanwhile, primary care physicians enable the bureaucracy to continue this expensive shell game as we continue our unheralded and significantly under-reimbursed work in the trenches—too busy to speak out against these injustices, too burdened by administrative obligations, and unable to afford the money or time to implement more creative ways to care for patients where they live.

When physicians and hospitals are "graded" on easy-to-measure outcomes that may or may not be clinically relevant—and are reimbursed only when complicated, often unpreventable bad outcomes don't occur—the incentive for health care enablers will be to weed out patients with any complicated illness or chronic condition and to care for only the young and healthy. Many physicians now limit their Medicare and Medicaid patient panels, sometimes refusing to see these patients at all. The sickest and most complicated patients will ultimately end up in safety net practices, like our residency program health centers, as increasingly hospital-employed and health system–employed practitioners compete for the healthiest and most compliant patients. When will the moral and financial incentives to provide high-quality, patient-centered care align meaningfully among physicians, hospitals, payors, and the public we serve?

I arrive at home at 5:17 p.m. The sun is just sneaking down past the trees, throwing shadows and reflections across the leaf litter. It's the glowing end of an Indian summer day. There's enough time to run.

Notes

1. Jordan Rau, "VA Experience Shows Patient 'Rebound' Hard to Counter," *Kaiser Health News* (September 12, 2011), http://www.kaiserhealthnews.org/Stories/2011/September/12/VA-readmissions.aspx

2. Camden Health Coalition, http://www.camdenhealth.org/

Calculating Caring

The small waiting room was packed with young mothers holding teary-eyed toddlers, older folks with resting tremors and oxygen tanks, and an obese man just stepping in from a smoke. I'm a family physician about to share my afternoon with each of them, in a working-class western Pennsylvania town. Walking quickly through the room on my way to the water cooler, I usually averted my gaze to avoid a not-so-private waiting room conversation with anyone. However, on this Wednesday afternoon, I stopped to stare at the television screen not silently suspended above a pregnant woman snuggling her sniffling son.

It was January 13, 2010. Haiti was imploding and crumbling in front of us, courtesy of CNN. Pictures of crushed bodies, partial glimpses of bloody limbs, and videos of screaming family members filled the screen. A steady stream of ticker-tape text gave up-to-the-moment information on the projected death toll, warnings of aftershocks, and reactions from around the globe. Descriptions like "natural war zone" did little to humanize the enormity of devastation unfolding before us.

Then the screen changed abruptly, faces of bantering politicians serving as a backdrop for the caption "Health Care Reform in Serious Jeopardy." These two stories were related somehow, but there was little time to reflect on their shared meaning as I left the waiting room to resume dealing with the afternoon's onslaught.

As the day dragged on, I became more distracted by thoughts of the immensity of the catastrophe in Haiti and increasingly moved by the efforts of hundreds of international volunteers who

101

were traveling to Haiti to help those trapped in the rubble. What motivated these health care workers and other professionals to put their own lives in danger to help others? Why did they care, and why should we? And why should we care about health care reform efforts' failing yet again, when polls tell us that so many Americans are "satisfied" with their health care plan?

Care Modifiers

I moved on through the afternoon, bothered by these questions as I addressed more immediate concerns. My daily menu of patient fare had not changed for years: folks suffering from inadequately controlled diabetes, emphysema worsened by ongoing cigarette smoking, depression partially managed with medications but not addressed by psychotherapy, and pregnancies complicated by high blood pressure. Patients with ear infections and abscesses that needed to be drained were added to spice up the day's schedule.

Using an electronic health record, touted as one of the cornerstones of efficiency and quality improvement for the health care system of the future, I dutifully recorded the care of my patients in medical shorthand. The data entered into these electronic records may one day help me improve the quality of care I deliver, but today the greatest accomplishment of this technology is to maximize billing and coding for patient care "services." The billing of medical services is a science unto itself—replete with rules, regulations, acronyms, and specialized lingo—and it demands a set of skills for which most doctors receive little formal training.

For instance, the fifty-seven-year-old diabetic patient with whom I spent twenty minutes discussing her inability to afford her sugar testing strips, her depression, and her failing marriage would be "coded" as a 99214 (designating her status as an "established" patient of "moderate complexity"). The computer program reminded me to add "modifiers" that would increase the billing and reimbursement I could obtain if the patient were fortunate enough to be insured. Discussing her alcohol use qualified for a modifier that paid me for counseling her to reduce the risks of alcohol abuse. Draining her abscess required another modifier that billed for the procedure itself.

Of course, the minutes spent scrolling through the various software panels and sifting through thousands of codes to submit this bill cost me precious patient care time. However, I am reminded by our practice manager that "if there is no margin, there is no mission"—referring to the financial sustainability we must maintain so that we can continue to deliver care, much of it not reimbursed, to the many patients in our practice who are uninsured or underinsured. Today more than 72 million Americans, nearly one out of every four of us, fall into this category.

As I finished the last appointment of the day and added the modifiers for the care I had delivered, I thought about the fundamental question of what motivates us to care for others—whether they be those who face overwhelming tragedy in a faraway land or those silently suffering in our own neighborhoods. As a primary care physician, I am incentivized professionally and financially to provide medically appropriate "care" for others. On a personal level, I care for others using a somewhat different set of modifiers and qualifiers, and I wonder about the mental mathematics that sum up my ability to care. Are there ways to incentivize people to care more for their neighbors, here or around the world?

Many people would find a picture of a suffering earthquake victim sufficiently compelling to move them to action—donating money, time, or talent. Fundraising experts know that depictions of single victims are often more effective at motivating people to care than images showing multiple victims, because the viewer feels less overwhelmed and more empowered to care for a smaller number of people. How powerful are "modifiers" to care related to numbers of victims, their location, or the cause of the devastation's being a natural disaster? A startling statistic from CNN flashes across the TV screen: 200,000 estimated dead under the rubble of Haiti. The sudden, unpredictable death and destruction contrasts with the estimated 205,000 lives lost in the United States due to lack of health insurance in the four-and-a-half years since Hurricane Katrina.

The Stories of Our Neighbors

This loss of life at home is no less devastating to me than the catastrophe in Haiti. Daily, I take care of patients who become these statistics, like the forty-eight-year-old construction worker and father of two with end-stage cancer diagnosed too late, after he couldn't afford to see doctors for over a year for his severe abdominal pain. Or the forty-six-year-old adult literacy teacher and father of three with coronary artery disease and poorly controlled diabetes, suffering with crushing chest pain and worsening heart problems because he can't afford his insulin and blood pressure medications.

Watching my patients sicken and die within the confines of our exclusionary, wasteful health care system makes me angry. What is even worse is that these patients have accepted with tired resignation that their lives have been cut short because they could not afford health care—demonstrating how thoroughly Americans have "bought" into the concept of health care as a discretionary commodity. How can I empower patients to care enough about changing our health care system, to demand more accountability and accessibility?

If only the personal narratives of these and many other similarly neglected patients were able to modify our willingness to care for others. These folks live among us and are our neighbors, coworkers, relatives, and friends. We could easily—by misfortune, accident, or untimely diagnosis—become one of them. But maybe their stories aren't dramatic enough.

Harrowing stories from Haiti, describing the devastation as a tragedy of biblical proportions, also depict heroic volunteers helping the wounded and grieving: physicians and nurses from around the globe performing life-saving amputations and surgeries around the clock and rescue workers lifting survivors buried beneath the crumbled remains of tenements and school buildings. A teenager pulled alive from the rubble after sixteen days is a powerful reminder of our extraordinary will to live. These accounts humanize and dramatize suffering and allow us to connect with others with whom we may have little in common except DNA. Their stories remind us that natural disasters, accidents, and medical catastrophes are equal-opportunity contingencies to which we are all vulnerable and that one day we too may need acts of common heroism to help us.

Even though the aftershocks have diminished, the devastation in Haiti continues because rebuilding and caring for the millions of displaced and disabled people will not happen quickly. Lacking a stable health care and political infrastructure and buried in poverty, thousands more Haitians will sicken and die unnecessarily in the coming months and years.

Unfortunately, a different lack of health care infrastructure exists in our country—despite annual spending of $2.7 trillion, or 17 percent of our gross domestic product (GDP), on health care. That half of all bankruptcies in the United States result from medical catastrophe is no surprise in light of a private health insurance system that denies coverage to people with preexisting conditions and spends more than thirty cents of every health care dollar on administrative overhead, rather than on health care delivery. The disparity between health care haves and have-nots is as striking as it is demoralizing.

On the same afternoon that I share a family's joy on behalf of an insured sixty-five-year-old patient of mine who received a heart transplant, I walk into the next room to discuss hospice plans with a fifty-two-year-old uninsured gentleman who had suffered silently for two years without medical attention for painful urinary tract problems, only to be diagnosed with end-stage prostate cancer. I see these stark contrasts in care and outcomes on a daily basis, but I can never accept them.

What Are the Costs of Care?

Many negative modifiers to care are insidious and buried in our subconscious, determining under what circumstances someone "deserves" care. What does caring cost me on an individual and societal level? The earthquake in Haiti exposed not only the fragility and evanescence of human enterprise but also the necessity of charitable responses driven by the motivation to "do the right thing." But when does the cost of doing right, of helping others, become too great?

Despite the current financial crisis, Americans have generously given hundreds of millions of dollars toward Haitian relief through federal grants and individual donations. Voices in opposition to this allocation of resources have been few. However, the debate on health care reform has highlighted a stern opposition among some politicians who argue that taxpayers shouldn't shoulder the burden of health care costs, which they say threatens to create a "socialized" system of medicine. How can we remind Americans that we all already pay for health care in this country—through our taxes, lower wages, and increasing individual contributions toward health insurance premiums, along with less state funding for public education as money is diverted to pay for Medicaid? Our failure to demand more quality, more accessibility, and less administrative waste from our taxpayer-funded health care system plays into the hands of those who are already profiting magnificently from this fragmented "system" of care. Don't we deserve better?

Perhaps we should really ask who deserves our care. People who are unemployed, receive welfare benefits, suffer from substance abuse, or are criminals or illegal aliens are often deemed undeserving of care, even deserving of bad outcomes. A recent letter by an emergency room physician questioned the "entitlement" of a poor, unemployed woman receiving Medicaid and food stamps because she had tattoos and smoked cigarettes. No doubt many Americans share the views this physician expressed about a culture of irresponsible spending, implicitly demanding a means test by which people who truly deserve care can be identified.

What about insured people who by accident of birth inherited fortunes and never had to work, who presided over financial scandals or benefited from environmental destruction or the exploitation of natural resources? Are they any more deserving of health care? Are they not also paradigmatic of a culture of irresponsibility?

Fortunately, religious and ethical considerations motivate us to be caring toward all of these individuals, even the most socially marginalized. How we judge others says a lot more about ourselves than about the subjects of our judgment. What do these modifiers tell us about our own values? As physicians who take an oath of responsibility, we are called on professionally to care, to set aside judgment, and to advocate in the best interests of our patients. Has our medical community forgotten these values? Or has the recitation of the Hippocratic Oath become a hollow exercise in sentimentality?

In primary care and psychiatry, we use a "harm reduction model" to care for patients with complicated medical and behavioral problems, striving to palliate their conditions and improve the quality of life for them and their families. Using a nonjudgmental approach, we acknowledge that a cure may not be possible, and we celebrate small victories with our patients—such as cutting down on tobacco use or losing a few pounds—empowering them to improve even though we don't expect perfection. We need to apply the same kind of pragmatic expectations to health care reform—focusing on the major themes of accessibility, cost control, and better quality of care—even as we expect that the process will be painful, like any necessary change.

The recently passed health care reform legislation is a significant first step toward increasing accessibility and ending deplorable market-driven private insurance tactics such as rescission. However, health care finance still needs substantial ongoing reform; with a growing and aging population, the proposed Medicare cuts will be powerful disincentives for physicians and hospitals to provide the quality care that patients of any age deserve. We still need to fundamentally restructure how we pay for health care, an issue that remains unaddressed. The addition of a public option would have enhanced competition among private insurance plans to cut unnecessary administrative costs, but its demise in the final negotiations that led to passage of the reform bill was an unfortunate concession to an insurance industry laden with conflicts of interest. Thoughtful consideration of a single-payer plan is still essential to the creation of a truly sustainable health care system.

Caring Is Good for All of Us

I'm moved by the outpouring of concern for the victims of the earthquake in Haiti because it demonstrates the caring, better side of our humanity. I'm disappointed by the ongoing public opposition to health care reform because it highlights the fearful, darker side of human nature. Despite economic and health policy evidence that supports the need for fundamental change in our health care system, many Americans seem unable to accept or embrace this momentous opportunity. Before passage of the reform legislation, cynics had claimed that moral arguments could not move the public to bring about meaningful, necessary change in our health care system. Out of fear of the unknown, we had settled for an established, inequitable, and wasteful present, with more than 45,000 people dying each year because of lack of health insurance. Now that we have taken an important first step, we need to continue our efforts to transform the system, to strive as a society toward a brighter future in which health care will be accessible to all and sustainable for years to come.

Why should we care about ongoing health care reform? And why should we continue to care about Haiti or—for that matter—the victims of recent earthquakes in Chile and China,

West Virginia coal miners crushed in cave-ins, or oil rig workers lost off the Louisiana coast? Because it is time to acknowledge the selfish part of caring: that we care for others because caring benefits us, too; that any altruistic act ultimately benefits the actor in some small way, and not just the beneficiary. Because in the end, we care for others knowing that we will need care from them in the future, on both an individual and a societal level. Confucius, Rabbi Hillel, Jesus, Muhammad, and secular humanists have all said it: we should treat others the way we would want them to treat us. We are all part of a larger community, and we bear responsibility for others in this fundamental act of connection.

We must realize that doing the right thing in health care, in Haiti or in these United States, is more than a human interest story. It is ultimately in our own best interest that health care be treasured as a human right and bestowed upon others as we would have it bestowed upon us.

Steep Sledding

"Don't worry," my doctor said.

I barely heard what he was saying; lying there in the hospital bed, I was caught up in contemplating the diagnostic procedure I was scheduled to have the next morning.

"With these anesthetics," he continued, "you won't feel or remember a thing after it's over."

"Okay," I answered weakly, signing the consent form with unaccustomed legibility. But could I really forget the emotional trauma of these past twelve hours?

I'm a physician and blessedly accustomed to standing on the other side of the health-and-illness divide. But after four days of crampy abdominal pain, my self-diagnosed "gastroenteritis" had horribly morphed into a "rule out carcinoma" directive. Now I faced another twelve hours of waiting—reviewing the possibilities, expecting the worst—until my procedure could be performed. Could I stop silently reviewing my CAT scan findings (that suspicious abdominal mass) and numb my feelings of anguish and anticipatory grief?

"Do you want a sleeping pill for tonight?" asked my doctor.

"I don't know," I stammered.

"It may help you sleep," he pressed.

"Okay," I said, grasping at the chance to escape this nightmare. Inwardly, though, I craved normal sleep, complete with dreams—not anesthesia's timeless, dreamless fugue state.

A brief visit from my wife and two young children helped me feel almost normal again. My wife Marilyn was supportive and ever hopeful as usual, telling me that she thought this was

110

still an infection. "Let's see what the test shows first, and we'll move on from there." However, it wasn't long before I returned to worrying about the possibility of our future together being cut terribly short.

Fortunately, my children distracted themselves and me by pointing out the vagaries of hospital bed controls. "Dad, wouldn't it be great to have a bed that moved like this at home?" my son Davey asked as the foot of the hospital bed went up and down.

The highlight, for me, was watching my seven-year-old daughter Grace skipping down the hospital hallway as she headed for the elevators to leave. Her carefree skipping was a precious invitation to forget my anxiety and enjoy the moment, and I did.

After they left, I endured two hours of cable TV cooking shows until the nurse finally brought in my benzodiazepine nightcap.

"This will never work," I thought, closing my eyes and tugging my stiff white sheets out of their hospital corners.

But I was wrong.

Half an hour later, it seemed, I found myself standing in my front yard in midwinter, staring down the small slope that led to the street. Grace, clad in snowsuit and red-striped stocking ski cap, smiled broadly at me as she mounted a sled.

"Don't worry," she told me. "It'll be all right."

Then she was off, squealing with delight as the snow swirled behind her and picking up speed as the hill somehow grew steeper and longer. She was heading for the street—and straight for our neighbor's house.

"Wait, stop!" I screamed. I ran down the hill, trying to keep her from getting hit by a car or plowing headfirst into our neighbor's front porch.

Instead, Grace accelerated, laughing all the way to the bottom. She hit a bump and started flying through the air.

I stood staring in disbelief and horror as she gained altitude, climbing impossibly high up over my neighbor's house and ancient hemlock tree, then dropping down and disappearing into their backyard, her striped ski cap a tiny flame flickering goodbye.

In a panic, I dashed behind the neighbor's house and found Grace.

She was making a snow angel. Snowflakes glistening on her nose, she cheerfully greeted me.

"That was fun! Let's do it again!"

"Okay," I said with relief.

Just then, the nurse tugged at my hospital gown.

"Wake up, it's time for your morning medications. They'll be taking you down for your procedure in a few minutes."

I looked around the hospital room. My IV was still running, the nurses' call button was still at my side, and the institutional green walls still needed a fresh coat of paint; but everything looked different somehow.

The same was true for me. I was still facing the same uncertainties and fears, but they didn't feel so terrible now. Something had shifted inside.

"All right," I replied. "I'm ready."

Minutes

Dutifully recorded,
respectfully submitted,
the minutes
reminded me that I had been there,
appearing engaged,
feigning thoughtfulness,
a room full of bobbleheads
wobbling toward consensus:

"Budget constraints,
robust analysis.
Abstracting, data mining,
breakout groups;
risk mitigation,
low-hanging fruit,
time constraints."

Minutes later
while wading through memos,
my tired patient called, who would rather be
clearing the breakfast dishes,
chauffeuring her teenage daughters,
secretly screening their Facebook accounts—
anywhere else, please,
but the necessary here, unscheduled:

"Going for chemo next week,
pain is bearable now;
my follow-up scan is in a month—
I may lose it if it's positive.
My husband's been a diamond in the rough;
this really isn't fair to him.
Thanks for listening."

I hung up the phone
and closed my eyes,
committing our conversation
to memory—

because there would be
no minutes
to rely on,

or at least
not enough.

Bereavement

"Suspended animation,"
said my seven-year-old son,
spying the streamlined apparition
barely resisting gravity
at the bottom of an aquarium.
"That nurse shark, he's
two hundred and sixty million years old."
Here was eternity at work,
cold efficiency revealed in
lidless eyes and
advantageously crafted
lack of conscience.

"Suspended animation,"
cried my grieving friend,
arriving at the home of her dearest companion,
finding the half-eaten dinner, cluttered rooms,
and framed smiling friends
silent with the promise of life ongoing,
the hoped-for momentary absence;
betrayed forever in her discovery
of his unblinking gaze
and quiet blue body
floating limply,
not at rest.

So heavy are these remains,
these truths we invested
in diaries and photographs,
petrified skeletons and fossilized teeth.
So weightless now
are those reasons,
religions, intuitions,
as I suspend my belief.

"Dad, he's moving,"
my son calls as he points to the aquarium.
I turn quickly to see for myself,
and the shark is gone.
"Don't worry," my son laughs.
"He'll be back."

In Line at the Maine Clam House

The line we're standing in,
as long as March is gray
and just as inviting,
begins with teenage couples
laughing like they wish they could,
winds through narrow-eyed
Harley-Davidson disciples
and out-of-towners adorned
in flip-flops and plaid shorts,
ends at the faded clapboard
menu outside Ken's Clam House.

You wouldn't believe
how comely a clam can be,
doused with beer and lightly battered,
after spending a lifetime filtering
God-knows-what on the ocean floor.

I wait in line to order clam bellies
for my son and daughter,
while my father, miles away,
prays over a hospital tray of damp potatoes
and half-baked cod.

My father speaks sparingly
of his past un-American;
though from his hospital bed he tells me
of his grandmother in Korea
who taught him about faith,
about gathering in pews,
purse-lipped women to the east
and stern-faced men to the west.
About how to sit in silence
for hours at a time,
apart, alone.

His grandmother dived for clams
using a knife with steely purpose,
deftly prying the clam
from its rocky hold,
scooping the soft gray-black belly
from the pearly inner shell,
and stirring the briny poached remains
to make a hungry child smile
and feel full with solitude,
nourished to withstand
transoceanic crossings
and cold stares.

I think of him now
as this line moves faster,
while my father, miles away,
goes under the knife,
towards another trackable outcome,
another crossing.

My son and daughter lean together,
and I step forward.
The waitress looks past me,
clicks her gum and beckons.
"Next in line, please."

Part 3
Jennifer Middleton, MD, MPH

I am Jen Middleton, the most junior of the group. I did my residency in family medicine at UPMC St. Margaret, and then I did a faculty development fellowship with Joel. It was during that time that Jon and Joel encouraged me to write. I stayed at St. Margaret to teach for another few years after that, but then I moved to Ohio in 2011.

Before I was a doctor, the stories that most caught my interest were the fanciful ones I imagined. I had been writing inconsequential fiction tales for many years before I graduated from medical school and headed to residency. The stories had never been more than a hobby for me, and I had never been brave enough to share them.

It was only in residency that I began writing nonfiction stories of my experiences with any regular frequency; it was only in residency that the emotion and power of my life stories began to rival the imagined ones of my youth. None of the narrative pieces that I wrote began life as planned pieces for publication. They were just stories that I couldn't get out of my head and that I needed to process—and the way that I had always processed events was to journal and write.

Still, it had never occurred to me to do anything with those pieces until I began to attend family medicine conferences. At those meetings, I discovered sessions on creative and formal medical writing. I met other people who were writing about the experience of being a physician. I learned that many of them were also publishing their work. Before these experiences, I had never considered that there might be an outlet for my writing.

I was fortunate to train for residency and fellowship in a program with an excellent tradition of supporting narrative writing. Jon Han and Joel Merenstein mentored my efforts, offering helpful feedback and suggestions on where to submit pieces for publication. Once I was brave enough to submit some pieces, I enjoyed some early successes, publishing a few narrative stories in family medicine journals.

Then the events of "Today I'm Grieving a Physician Suicide" happened. I wrote the earliest draft of that piece without any intention to publish; again, the need to process and expel the heavy swirl of internal emotion was my only motivation. Some unnamed need to vent my anger compelled me to share the piece with Joel and Jon, and their encouragement led me to submit it for publication. The wise editors at the *Annals of Family Medicine* pushed me to include a brief review of the medical literature on physician suicide, and as a result, I learned that I could use my individual narrative to advocate for change. Writing about difficult times like that one has helped me to better understand my own truths.

I first learned about medical blogging at another regional family medicine conference. I learned, also, about Twitter and the incredible depth of medical writing and thought generating that happen behind the scenes of those 140-character posts. The opportunity to advocate for family medicine and share my stories in this new format was too tempting to pass up, and The Singing Pen of Doctor Jen was born.

Blogging is very different from submitting to journals! There are no editors or peer review, just a few paragraphs of my thoughts posted every few days. Writing for a blog is also very different from preparing a narrative piece for publication. I have a "one hour" rule to keep myself from the lure of endless revision; I allow myself only sixty minutes from the time I start writing a post to when I publish it. This rule keeps my posts short and focused, and it also preserves their rawness and energy. Though I remove all traces of identifying information before sharing issues related to the patients and residents I interact with, hopefully my readers are getting an authentic glimpse into the life of a residency educator.

The blog posts that I've included here stand in significant contrast to the more polished essays that precede them. The time and care that goes into crafting an elegant and meaningful personal essay produces valuable and deeply insightful pieces; blogs, on the other hand, allow the opportunity to share a longitudinal dialogue with readers, where the themes and story arcs that develop over time happen organically and without conscious planning.

The positive energy on Twitter and the blogosphere is overwhelming; I never would have guessed that a virtual space could be so affirming. Between the blog and Twitter, I have "met" many new friends and colleagues. By sharing comments on each other's posts and forwarding each other's tweets, we offer encouragement, new ideas, and support to each other. I've found that I desperately need that affirmation. As a young attending and junior faculty member, I was constantly questioning my actions—and today, the consequences of many of the kinds of decisions I have to make (for patients and learners alike) can be serious and far-reaching, leading to a heavy and unprecedented burden of responsibility.

I recently celebrated my ten-year medical school reunion, and as I move into the middle of my career, I am perhaps a bit more comfortable about being a physician—though I still fear that I will never truly quell my day-to-day anxieties. Writing through these uncertainties helps me to process my thoughts and reach a deeper level of understanding about my experiences. As I progress through my career, the context within which I now see my previous pieces seems to get increasingly broad and more universal.

In this book, I have included published stories, unpublished stories, and a collection of posts from my blog. Although technology has given my generation new avenues to share our ideas, it's the sharing itself that will always remain most important. The act of writing forces me to find the words to explain feelings and ideas that would otherwise remain ill defined and unheard. I've come to know myself better by writing through the challenges I've experienced, and this process has helped me to both live a more authentic life and connect more authentically with others.

Today I'm Grieving a Physician Suicide

Today I learned that you died, and nothing will ever be the same again. I refused to believe the words I heard, that you committed suicide. Only terribly depressed people kill themselves. You weren't terribly depressed . . . but then I learned that yes, secretly you had been. How could I not know, not realize?

Your body will be laid to rest in three days. My body doesn't seem to belong to me anymore—it walks and talks, it swallows food and gets in the shower, but it's as if my mind has flown above it so that I can't feel the gut-wrenching agony threatening to consume me.

Why didn't you ask your physician colleagues for help? Why did you hide your depression from us? Did I, as your colleague and friend, fail you? These questions circle relentlessly through my mind. I need to understand, need somehow for this all to make sense.

• • •

Today I'm struggling with the awkward conversations regarding your death. "I would have helped if I had only known," so many said. Did you fear losing the respect of your colleagues and coworkers if they had indeed known? The culture of medicine demands that physicians suppress vulnerability or need,[1,2] and this ethos does not accept help-seeking behavior.[3] A recent JAMA Consensus Statement concluded that the stigma against physicians

125

with depression is a strong disincentive for obtaining treatment.[4] I worry that this "macho mentality"[5] of medicine may have dissuaded you from confiding your suicidal thoughts to anyone.

I knew you as both my colleague and my friend. Your spirit is still the most generous and insightful I have ever known. Your smile was bright and full of compassion. You shared your opera tickets with me and listened simply to my insecurities. You brought a bakery cake and candles to my birthday dinner at a local restaurant last year and led the table in singing to me.

Everyone keeps asking whether I'm OK. What am I supposed to say? I lie most of the time. I figure that they would rather hear platitudes than the truth. The bitterly frigid vestiges of winter's finale cut into my coat and pierce my skin. Everything is too bright, too cold, too sterile.

· · ·

Today I learned the details of your death. I thought about writing them here; I want to see the words blazing out at me. I want the page to groan from the pain of your last days and hours. I want it to cry out, "Enough! How can we let this keep happening?"

I realized, however, that it does keep happening. Depression is as common among physicians as it is in the general population, and we commit suicide at higher rates.[6] Some of that difference may be explained by both our knowledge about and our access to lethal means,[7] but that explanation is incomplete. Overall, most doctors hesitate to address depression in both themselves and their colleagues.[8] This fact is unsurprising considering how our professional culture stigmatizes depression. A physician who survived a suicide attempt asked, "Do we as doctors accept depression as a treatable medical illness—as long as the patient isn't one of us?"[9] I choose to reject any assertion that your death was the result of some fundamental weakness or personality flaw; I see no dishonor in either the manner of your death or of the disease process that led you there.

The JAMA Consensus Statement on physician depression and suicide was published in 2003, almost four years before you died. What, if anything, has changed in that time? I am frustrated by our profession's resigned acceptance of your death. Individually, we wring our hands in frustration and wonder how we might have intervened, but collectively I see no concerted effort to address this problem. I feel alone in my indignation and anger.

. . .

Today I tasted food for the first time since your death. It's as though my mind has gotten brave enough to exist inside my body again. I can feel the rebound of the keys as I type, can hear the quiet hum of the desk lamp's bulb beside me. I keep the television on, barely loud enough to hear, its delicate river of noise flowing behind me. I need those dim, purposeless amplitudes, need anything more than just my thoughts for company; it's too unbearable to cycle through my memories and the pieced-together imaginings of your final day.

I wonder whether we, whether I, missed the signs of your impending suicide. Studies in the 1970s and 1980s described the physician at high risk of suicide as driven, competitive, and compulsive;[10] having few friends[11] and no spouse;[12] and most importantly, having a history of depression or substance abuse.[13] You were certainly hardworking and diligent, but those traits hardly distinguish you from most other physicians. You had a sizable social network. You were receiving mental health care before you died, but few of us surrounding you knew, as you did not disclose your depression diagnosis to anyone but your closest friends and family. I am left contemplating what share of the responsibility, of the guilt, should be mine.

Sleep remains elusive for me, nothing more than short intervals of dreamless stupor interspersed with endless stretches of the clock face's screaming inanity. Did you sleep the night before you died?

• • •

Today a visiting lecturer commented that 250 physicians commit suicide every year in the United States.[14] Hearing that number knocks the breath out of me. Two hundred fifty souls who will lose their battle with the dark, cognitive distortions of depression. Two hundred fifty populations of families, classmates, friends, and colleagues whose lives will be forever scarred.

How many others in my life are suffering silently, as you did? I thought I knew you, understood you, but clearly I didn't really know you at all. My intuition will now be forever suspect. I realize that I have been scripting the lives of those around me according to my own understandings and experiences instead of allowing their unique truths to touch me.

I'm less concerned with getting to the diagnosis and plan in my patient encounters now, as I'm suddenly much more interested in my patients' stories. I find myself listening more intently to what they say to me, searching for clues to their words' intended meaning, prompting them to share more. I have always wanted to ease suffering as a physician, but I never understood what the depths of that suffering could be before. I do not think that my treatment goals themselves have changed, but I hope that my interactions with patients now express better the depths of my concern for them and my genuine desire to understand them as individuals.

• • •

As the months have passed, the acute pain of your loss has dulled, but the questions remain. Why didn't you ask for help? Why did you hide your depression? Did I, as your colleague and friend, fail you? Despite my exploration of the literature, I can still only speculate at the answers. I have no doubt, however, that we cannot continue to neglect the issue of physician suicide.

Two hundred forty-nine other physicians will commit suicide this year. This number indicates no less than an ongoing crisis, yet I have found that few researchers have studied physician suicide, and what little literature does exist is mostly outdated.[12] Increasing attention to this devastating problem may encourage dialog among physicians, perhaps decreasing the shame surrounding our mental health issues and creating collaboration to find solutions. All of us as physicians also have a responsibility to contribute to a professional culture that, instead of stigmatizing and isolating, is affirming and supportive.

I wonder how many more physicians' lives will be lost before we confront this silent crisis of depression and suicide in our profession; I can only wish that we might start today.

Acknowledgment

The author wishes to acknowledge the kind assistance of Ms. Joann Buckley; Jonathan Han, MD; and Joel Merenstein, MD.

Notes

1. Claudia Center et al., "Confronting Depression and Suicide in Physicians: A Consensus Statement," *Journal of the American Medical Association* 289, no. 23 (2003): 3161–66.

2. Merry N. Miller and K. Ramsey McGowen, "The Painful Truth: Physicians Are Not Invincible," *Southern Medical Journal* 93, no. 10 (2000): 966–73.

3. Miller and McGowen, "The Painful Truth."

4. Center et al., "Confronting Depression and Suicide in Physicians."

5. Miller and McGowen, "The Painful Truth."

6. Center et al., "Confronting Depression and Suicide in Physicians"; Miller and McGowen, "The Painful Truth"; Dario

M. Torre et al., "Suicide Compared to Other Causes of Mortality in Physicians," *Suicide and Life-Threatening Behavior*, 35, no 2 (2005): 146–53; D. Black, "When Physicians Commit Suicide," *Iowa Medicine: Journal of the Iowa Medical Society*, 82, no 2 (1992): 58–61; Victor M. Victoroff, "My Dear Colleague: Are You Considering Suicide?" *Journal of the American Medical Association* 254, no 24 (1985): 3464–66; Herbert Hendin, John T. Maltsberger, and Ann Pollinger Haas, "A Physician's Suicide," *The American Journal of Psychiatry* 160, no 12 (2003): 2094–97.

7. Black, "When Physicians Commit Suicide."

8. Center et al., "Confronting Depression and Suicide in Physicians."

9. Gayleen M. Eilers, "I Was a Success at Everything—Except Suicide," *Wisconsin Medical Journal* 95, no 4 (1996): 223–25.

10. Center et al., "Confronting Depression and Suicide in Physicians"; Miller and McGowen, "The Painful Truth."

11. Miller and McGowen, "The Painful Truth."

12. Center et al., "Confronting Depression and Suicide in Physicians."

13. Center et al., "Confronting Depression and Suicide in Physicians"; Miller and McGowen, "The Painful Truth"; Black, "When Physicians Commit Suicide."

14. Tom Schwenk (lecture, UPMC St. Margaret, Pittsburgh, PA, June 2007).

Fallibility/Forgiveness

Mr. Green (all names, except mine, have been changed) was elderly, with end-stage lymphoma and an intelligent, diligent wife.

"Something's not right with him," she told me in the Emergency Department (ED). "I was a nurse for a long time, and I can't tell you what it is, but something is wrong." Her hair was neatly permed, her blue blouse meticulously ironed.

I was a family medicine intern, slogging through a weekend call shift. My hair was sloppily pulled back by bobby pins, and my scrubs were wrinkled and ill fitting. I looked at my new patient, and he smiled wanly at me.

"How do you feel?"

"Tired," his voice simultaneously full of fatigue and kindness. "But I just had another round of chemo yesterday." He is momentarily dyspneic after uttering this short sentence.

As his wife begins to tell his story and I begin to scribe it, my pager goes off.

Beep beep beep beep.

I silence the pager, making a mental note to answer it once she's finished.

"He keeps getting so short of breath," she exclaims.

Beep beep beep beep.

I hit the silence button again. "I'm sorry, please continue."

She seems unruffled by the electronic invasions. "And he hasn't really been hungry for a few days."

Beep beep beep beep.

She touches me on the arm. "Go ahead and answer it, honey. We're not going anywhere."

I apologetically excuse myself and step out to the phone in the ED hallway.

I return the first page. "Are you done yet?" barks my senior resident from the phone's receiver.

"Uh, no, I only just got to this one."

"Which one?"

"Mr. Green, the seventy-three-year-old with lymphoma."

"The cancer guy with the dwindles?" He sounds harried, and I can hear his pager going off as if he were sitting next to me instead of standing somewhere four floors away. "Just get him an IV and consult oncology—we're down seven admissions already."

I like Mr. and Mrs. Green, but my intern confidence is still too shaky to let anything override my senior's exhortation. I pull the curtain back, sit down, take a hasty review of systems, perform a perfunctory exam, and exit the room. I finish scrawling my H&P, start writing my orders, and place my call to the attending.

The attending, Dr. Brennon, calls back promptly.

"I'm afraid I don't have a good explanation for his tachycardia and renal failure besides dehydration, Dr. B," I conclude hesitantly. "I can't find anything else in his exam or EKG or labs to explain it."

"Well, chemo can definitely tire people out." Dr. Brennon's bright voice sounds slightly tinny and far away. "Let's see if we can tank him up overnight, and I'll see him first thing in the morning."

I hang up and glance at my wristwatch: 8:53 p.m. I automatically do the arithmetic—10 hours, 7 minutes left in my call shift. I turn to my almost finished orders.

"Code blue, 561. Code blue, 561. Code blue, 561," calls the operator calmly overhead.

Mr. Green's orders would have to wait; I slam down my pen and sprint for the stairs. "Shoot those orders upstairs, will you? I'll finish them later!" I shout at the ED nurse.

The night continued on in a frenzied blur of activity. I did get back to Mr. Green's chart upstairs to scribble the rest of his orders, but his nurse called me in the middle of my eighth admission for the shift two hours after that.

"Dr. Middleton, I think you forgot to write fluid orders for this patient."

"I'm sorry, it's been so crazy." My pager is going off again, and my lips recite the verbal order automatically: "Half-normal saline with 20 of K at 100 an hour."

He "code yellowed" three hours later. "Code yellow" in our hospital is a designation for the abruptly crumping patient who is in imminent danger of becoming a code blue. The call team—me, another intern, and our senior—rushed to his side.

"What's this guy's story again?" yells my senior over the hubbub. Mr. Green is slumped, unresponsive, in his hospital bed. He is febrile, and his breath comes in shallow gasps.

"Lymphoma, 'dwindles,'" I remind him.

"Right. Well, he may be approaching septic now."

"To the unit?" I ask.

"Nah," says my senior. "His pressure's still okay, and he's satting okay. Let's start some antibiotics and put him on 3B." 3B is our cardiac monitor unit, literally just a few steps away from the ICU. I write the orders, answer Mrs. Green's questions, and get back to work.

I wearily pass my pagers off to the new call team as 7:00 a.m. finally arrives. Something about Mr. Green is nagging at me, though, and I head back to 3B to check on him. Even from the doorway, I can see that he is a shadow of the man I met barely 11 hours ago.

I see the attending sitting at the 3B nursing unit as I leave his room. "Dr. B? This guy needs to go to the unit." I launch into a rambled narrative of the night's events.

As I finish my litany, Dr. Brennon is nodding his head. "I agree."

"I'll write the orders," I offer.

We start working on it together when the operator's voice sounds overhead.

"Code blue, 351. Code blue, 351. Code blue, 351."

It's Mr. Green.

We bolt in and are greeted by the new call team.

"Jen? Go home," my freshly arrived intern colleague says. "We got this."

"No!" I protest. "I admitted him. I know him."

Meanwhile, Mrs. Green is tugging at my sleeve. "Doctor, should he have potassium in his IV fluids?"

A horrible, queasy, sinking feeling pummels into my gut. Everything suddenly fits—this man coded from a cardiac arrthymia. He has a cardiac arrhythmia because his potassium is too high. His potassium is too high because I put potassium into the IV fluid of a man with acute renal failure. The bag of saline is only inches away from my face as I push my way up to his bedside, and it seems to be sneering at me mockingly.

A nurse steers his wife out of the room. Somehow, in the chaos, I manage to inform the new on-call senior of my mistake. He shrugs, and I take my turns pounding on my patient's chest while he is intubated and bagged.

Thirty minutes later, the senior calls the code.

I stumble out of the room into the hallway. My exhaustion crumbles what little self-composure I have left, and I can't stop the tears. As I begin to shake, I feel arms around me. First it's one of the kindly 3B nurses, then she gives way for my resident colleagues. The three of them envelop me, overlapping me in a cocoon of safety as I sob uncontrollably.

"I killed him. I killed him. I killed him." It comes out in staccato gasps.

"Jen, he had advanced lymphoma, he was septic." My senior's voice. "You said so yourself."

"The potassium killed him. I killed him."

Dr. Brennon extricates me from them and steers me into an empty room. He sits, patiently, as I sniffle and repeatedly blow my nose.

"Jen, Dr. Schantz told them three weeks ago that he only had two weeks to live."

This statement doesn't help. "It doesn't matter, I killed him. I killed him, and his wife knows it."

Dr. Brennon considers this carefully. His words are careful, gentle, and measured. "You need to talk to her."

I know on some primal level that he's right, but an equally primal fear responds.

"I can't."

"Go in there and talk to her. Trust me."

I surrender my fear to my instructor's faith. I walk down the hall and enter his room.

She is sitting in a chair next to his bed. The nurses have already cleaned up all of the detritus from the code. The ET tube is still clamped in his mouth, though.

She sees me come in.

"I'm so sorry," I blurt out, hovering awkwardly in the doorway.

"It's not your fault," she says. She motions for me to come in; astounded at this welcome, I numbly stagger over to her. "I didn't want to believe Dr. Schantz. I know he's been our doctor for years and years, but I didn't want to believe him."

I sit on the floor next to her chair. She takes my hand.

"We've been married over fifty years," she continues. "He was just talking to me, just a few hours ago. How can he be gone?"

I have a burning need for her absolution, but I am too ashamed to ask for it. Besides, it seems terribly wrong to interrupt her; I do not fit inside her grief.

"You're so young," she observes. "How old are you?"

"Tw-tw-twenty-eight," I manage to stammer.

"It's so wonderful to see young women these days being doctors. In my day, we had to settle for being nurses. Not that nursing isn't noble, mind you. But it was our only choice." With her left hand, she is still holding my hand. With her right hand, she is smoothing his hair.

I let my tears fall onto the concrete floor, which is hard under me.

"You mustn't feel badly," she says. Her voice is quiet, calm, and dignified. "I knew the potassium might be a problem—I remembered that you said his kidneys weren't working very well—but I couldn't seem to say anything to the nurse about it."

My head remains bowed. The tiled floor has an oddly mesmerizing pattern.

"But it doesn't matter. It was his time. I appreciate you being honest about it."

She didn't let go of my hand, so I sat there with her for the next thirty minutes or so. It didn't seem right to get up and leave, and selfishly, I didn't want to break my connection with them. I remember the cold tile seeping through my scrubs; the salty taste of my tears; and her calm, resigned expression. I remember the way her silent tears splashed onto her blue blouse, leaving little wet stains.

She finally let go of my hand when the nurse entered to announce that their son was on his way.

Mrs. Green looked at me with determination. "I don't want him to see his father like this." She motioned to the ET tube.

I probably should have said that the tube had to stay in until he got to the morgue, that no one was allowed to pull them out after a code. Out loud, she verified that she, too, knew this fact, but the tone of her voice clearly indicated her intentions to override it. Both in awe of her composure and beholden to her clemency, I grabbed a couple of washcloths from the bathroom while she unstrapped the ET tube holder. Newly confident, I gently gripped the ET tube with a washcloth. Her hands rested over mine. "Let me do it. That way, you won't get in trouble." Not possessing the will to protest, I stepped away, and in one smooth motion she removed the tube and laid it at the bedside. I wiped his mouth with another washcloth. We straightened the bedsheets. She lifted his head while I repositioned his pillow. We stood there, co-conspirators and allies, nodding our approval to each other.

The son appeared in the doorway and went straight to his mother's arms. I suddenly felt superfluous, and I quietly slipped out of the room as they turned to the bedside of Mr. Green. I could rationalize about his terminal condition, his sepsis. I could say with some truth that he probably would have died anyway, even if I had ordered the correct IV fluids.

But he died at the moment and in the manner that he did because of me. That is my truth, a truth I will carry with me for the rest of my career and beyond. If there is meaning in it beyond my fallibility, beyond his wife's incredible capacity for forgiveness and grace, beyond my classmates' unconditional acceptance, then it is beyond my comprehension. Those alone will provide a lifetime's worth of meaning for me.

Acknowledgment

The author wishes to acknowledge the kind assistance of Jonathan Han, MD, and Joel Merenstein, MD, in preparing this story.

Our Family Doctor

I met the Johnsons (not their real name) toward the end of my intern year, when I was still trying to figure out how to be a doctor. In their early fifties, they were everything I was not: vibrant, eloquent, and confident.

"No real problems, doc," William told me in his deep baritone. "Just this gallbladder cancer, but I think we've got that licked."

Margaret nodded, resting a hand on his arm. "The cancer doctors told us he wouldn't have long to live, but he feels so well now after the surgery."

I consulted the chart. *Cholangiocarcinoma*, three months status post-resection. I looked at their hopeful faces, which clashed with everything my medical knowledge base told me about his disease. Their beaming countenances contradicted my education; they believed that he was going to be OK. I couldn't find the words to tell them that his prognosis was terribly poor.

"We just bought a new truck—we saved for ten years to buy that truck," William said. He certainly looked well—neatly dressed, vigorous, proud face shining. This image of cancer did not fit with my medical training to date at all. Their surety agitated my already tenuous intern confidence. I managed to mumble something about keeping up with his oncology appointments, all the while envying their faith in life's goodness.

By this point in the intern year of my family medicine residency, I was exhausted—physically, mentally, and spiritually. Ten months before, I had graduated from medical school with a level of enthusiasm that was almost certainly obnoxiously grating to the experienced physicians around me. But now, as my intern year was ending, I couldn't believe that I had ever once had so much faith in myself and in our profession. Our failures assaulted me daily. I constantly second-guessed my decision to turn my life over to this monster that demanded more of my soul than I wanted to give up. I wondered why I couldn't believe the way Margaret and William Johnson did.

• • •

Three months have passed. William is now in the Intensive Care Unit at St. Margaret, admitted earlier in the week with fever and belly pain. His condition has rapidly deteriorated, and tonight he is on a vent and two pressors, dying of septic shock. I'm not assigned to the ICU this month, but I stop by to check up on him. I look over today's CT scan—his abdomen is full of cancer. I look at the monitors and the labs, unsatisfied.

I walk into his room and sit next to him. The monitors click and beep softly around us as tinted liquids ooze through multiple IVs. His face contorts into odd grimaces, but the sedation and ET tube prevent him from sharing the details of his personal agony. Even this early into my training, I recognize the scene before me. This image of cancer does fit with my medical knowledge base, and a new, eerily confident realization settles into my gut.

"He's going to die tonight."

"I think you're right," a voice responds.

I turn around; I hadn't realized I had spoken the thought out loud. Debbie, one of our best ICU nurses, has entered the room.

"I thought I saw you come in here," she says.

I turn to her, my novice's eyes begging her to contradict me.

"He's going to die," she says.

The *whrrrs* of the ventilator punctuate this sentence for me.

"The family's coming in to discuss withdrawing care," Debbie tells me gently. "They'll be glad to know you're here."

I feel the weight of responsibility. The family's going to expect me to help them decide. Will they leave the decision about his life support up to me? Who am I to help decide such things?

I look at him again.

Nothing I can do or say will save his life. I grit my teeth; Margaret has insisted repeatedly during the past week that we "do everything—Willie's going to beat this." But the end has come, heedless of any of our wishes. My newfound confidence asserts itself again. It's not my responsibility to help them decide if he keeps on living; it's my job to help him die well.

The conversation with Margaret is difficult. I start out talking the way I think a doctor should talk. "His condition is failing. We can't do anything to change what's going to happen."

But I know this family now, and the generic words sound hollow and staid. I switch gears and talk to Margaret as I would my own family. "What would Willie want, Margaret?"

Tears are streaming down her cheeks. "He's ready to go; I know he is. I'm just not ready."

I nod my head. "Call the rest of the family in." A phrase comes to mind that I have heard the ICU nurses say many times. "We'll give him a beautiful death."

And we do. At least a dozen members of William Johnson's family gather outside the ICU while Debbie and I extubate him, disconnect his IVs, and pull all of the poles and ventilation equipment out of the room. We put a fresh gown on him and a clean blanket on his bed. We drag in every spare chair and box of tissues we can find.

I go out to get the family from the waiting room, but I don't need to introduce myself.

"This is Dr. Middleton," says Margaret firmly. "She's our doctor."

The family murmur and nod approvingly as I digest the import of her statement. Up until this moment, I haven't been used to thinking of myself as a doctor, let alone a doctor that belonged to anyone, to a family.

"We're ready for you to come back now. You can sit with him, talk to him, hold his hand even, if you like." I repeat the mantra I have heard Debbie give families so many times, struggling to keep my voice steady and composed as I blink away tears. I wonder if real doctors are supposed to cry with their families.

I lead them back into the room, its curtains respectfully lining the windows. Margaret sits in the chair Debbie has specifically placed next to Willie, on the side with the hand and wrist unmarred by multiple arterial line attempts. She takes his hand. "Can he hear me?"

I swallow and tell the truth, or at least my truth. "I believe he can. I believe he's waiting for you to give him permission to go."

Her daughter hands her a tissue, and Margaret struggles to find her voice. "I think you're right," she whispers to me. Her family nods their encouragement. She turns to her husband. "Willie, I love you. It's OK for you to go now. I'm going to be OK. You don't have to suffer anymore."

Debbie has a vial of morphine ready to inject in case Mr. Johnson shows any signs of pain or air hunger. We don't end up needing it, though. William Johnson dies quietly within the hour, surrounded by his children, grandchildren, and siblings, with his wife tenderly holding his hand.

$$\bullet \quad \bullet \quad \bullet$$

Over five years later, I still have the privilege of caring for Margaret Johnson, who continues to proclaim that I am her family's doctor. I used to think that patients belonged to doctors, but I know better now. I will always belong to them. I am, indeed, the Johnsons' doctor.

Acknowledgment

The author wishes to acknowledge the kind assistance of Jonathan Han, MD, and Joel Merenstein, MD, in preparing this manuscript.

A Eulogy to
My Former Self

Former Self, you have only been gone a few months, but already I find it difficult to remember you. What I still remember best are your incontrovertible beliefs. The present and its misery didn't matter, and a bright, shiny, faraway future beckoned on the other side. Time belonged to you, to divide and subdivide into tasks and obligations, and your destiny was completely under your control.

You expected friends and family to accept second-place position and priority, expected them to suffer your absence as you suffered theirs. After all, no profession could be nobler than yours—than medicine. You decided to cram a two-year fellowship and graduate degree program into thirteen months. You accepted additional time commitments without hesitation because they would bolster your CV. Rushing was the norm; anything less than a frenzied pace was for the weak.

Your body had no needs more important than work. The body was always a hindrance, anyway; its incessant demands for food and sleep were wastes of time. Your rational mind was separate and superior to these mundane bodily requirements. As for emotions, well, you carefully relegated them to an inaccessible place, apparently knowing on some subconscious level the threat they posed to your carefully arranged reality.

And then, one afternoon, everything stopped.

. . .

Stop.

Pain. Gnawing pain, just behind my left temple.

Partial visual loss on the left, a strange fracture across the left lower corner of my vision.

Fear.

The list of differential diagnoses starts to chime, unbidden, from years of educational indoctrination. CVA. Cavernous sinus thrombosis. Retinal artery occlusion. Optic nerve compression secondary to a mass. Optic neuritis.

Mentally, I sort them in order of likelihood as I sit on a stretcher in my hospital's Emergency Department.

I'm not supposed to be on this side of the curtain.

An hour later, I lie motionless on the cold, unforgiving slab of the MRI machine, willing my left eye to give up its secret. I am still ticking through my differential. I know what's at the top, given my age (thirty), my gender (female), my birthplace (northern latitude), and the season of my birth (winter). Another hour passes, and the ED physician returns to announce, "It's optic neuritis." I tell myself I'm not surprised, but it's still a shock.

I'm not supposed to be the patient.

Images of the debilitated women I've cared for with MS start flashing through my mind. I can see them distinctly, withered silent shapes swallowed up by the voluminous sheets of their hospital beds as their caregivers offer proxied histories.

The nurse comes in and asks, "Are you OK?" I know this ED nurse well. She's one of the really, really good ones. She's taken my orders for patients a thousand times before.

She's not supposed to be cradling me as I weep, sitting here in this stupid flimsy hospital gown. She knows what I know, what I conceal from most of my nonmedical friends and family when I eventually share this saga with them. She knows that optic neuritis most commonly occurs as a precursor to multiple sclerosis. She knows that I could, someday, become one of those crippled women.

She knows that my life has changed forever.

I get round one of a thousand milligrams IV methylprednisolone and agree to return to the outpatient medical unit tomorrow for round two. Round one, however, just made me vomit into one of those teeny pink plastic emesis basins, and I begin to realize just what I'm in for. I get some IV promethazine, and I go home to days and weeks of appointments and tests.

I will have long stretches of time to pass as my optic nerve heals, during which the massive doses of steroids will leave me restless and nauseated. I will discover that I cannot read, watch television, or look at a computer screen for more than ten minutes without a headache. Unable to escape into my usual realms of oblivion, I will ultimately spend this time questioning everything that I once held to be immutable in my life. Little that I recognize will remain afterward.

• • •

Former Self, I miss your fearlessness. Even months later, with my vision restored and a negative lumbar puncture behind me, I cannot rekindle that sense of power. When I listen to my patients, their vulnerabilities now resonate in my soul.

The specter of MS is a constant undercurrent, but not with the negative connotation you would have ascribed to it. You would have seen a threat to your well-ordered machinations. I consider it an insistent reminder about the value of the present—of living a rich, full life every moment of every day. I have learned that in the space of a heartbeat, everything can change forever. I still get overwhelmed thinking about the infinite number of those forevers and their possibilities.

So I bid you a bittersweet farewell. You were so powerful that nothing less than four weeks of imposed reflection could negate you. Your constant fight against a universe that continues its destiny heedless of your will, though, ultimately destroyed you. In your place, I instead surrender to possibility and unknowing, to faith and now.

I taste food carefully. My eyes marvel at the colors surrounding me, at the incredible variety of greens and blues and reds. I wake well rested to comfortably full days. My newly strengthened muscles enjoy scrambling over muddy tree-lined trails. Without shame, I laugh and share and cry and love.

Rest in peace, Former Self. Without you, I never would have arrived here, and here is a very fine place to be just now.

Selected posts from
"The Singing Pen of Doctor Jen" blog
http://singingpendrjen.blogspot.com

Thursday, January 27, 2011

A Paper Cut
in a Digital World

As I mentally gear up for another week on the inpatient team with our residents, I am vividly remembering a moment from my last week there.

First, a little background. About five years ago, our hospital went live with an electronic medical record. True, the documenting system is a bit clunky, but inputting daily progress notes, H&Ps, consults, and discharge summaries electronically became possible.

As a third-year resident here, I practically leaped for joy. Gone would be the days of squinting to read Dr. Scribbler's illegible H&P! Gone would be the days of hunting down a paper chart to read a consult! I imagined a beautiful new word of efficient legibility.

The majority of the attending staff, as you are probably already imaging, did not share my optimism. They were unhappy with the clunkiness I alluded to above. They didn't want to take the time to log in, pull up the right patient, open a new progress note, and type in their thoughts. "Too many clicks" became their

146

mantra. The hospital decided to continue allowing paper documentation while the IT folks worked on ways to make physician documentation less cumbersome and more user-friendly.

Fast-forward to my time on service last month. After a lengthy search, I had finally grabbed hold of a patient's paper chart. As I flipped through the pages to read the surgeon's recommendations for our patient, I felt a familiar sting in my index finger. A drop of blood welled onto the page I was reading.

Paper cut. I got a paper cut reading a patient's chart. Carpal tunnel from clicking the mouse too much? OK. Eyestrain from staring at LCD screens for too long? Understandable. But a paper cut?!?

It is 2011, and my hospital is still using a hybrid electronic-paper system. We are far from the only hospital still relying on paper this late into the twenty-first century. In all fairness, electronic documentation for physicians does need to become more intuitive and less cumbersome. But the time has come for us to demand better software, not go back and bury our heads in the sharp edges of an outmoded paper system. Resisting better legibility and faster data retrieval denies patients the accurate and timely medical documentation—and care—that they deserve.

Anybody got a Band-Aid?

What Ever Happened to "Doctor"?

I was sitting next to a resident in the preceptor room yester-
day. He was calling a patient to discuss lab results, and he introduced himself on the phone by his first name and last name...but
not with "Doctor." (e.g., "Hi, this is John Smith from the Family
Health Center.")

I occasionally see the residents' patients for urgent visits.
When I ask them who their regular PCP is at the office, I get a
first name response about half of the time (e.g., "Jane" or "Dr.
Jane"). I have seen this same phenomenon in the hospital when
I'm on the inpatient service; I'll reference the family medicine
resident caring for a particular patient by title and last name, and
the patient will say, "Who?" I have since learned to then provide
the resident's first name, to which the patient will invariably sigh
with relief and say, "Oh yes. He/she has been so nice."

You have probably guessed by now how I feel about this
use of first names. I may be only in my mid-thirties, but perhaps
I belong to an earlier era. I address my patients (over the age of
eighteen) by their titles and last names unless they have given
me permission to do otherwise. When I meet new patients, I
address them by their first and last names and then ask them how
they would like for me to address them. My expectation is that
they will address me as I prefer to be professionally addressed:
"Dr. Middleton."

I suspect the blurring of casual and corporate that has
occurred in the rest of the business world is happening in medi-

cine. I am addressed by my first name in the vast majority of transactions I undertake as a customer, almost always by people who don't know me. Perhaps the "Doctor" title is yet another casualty of that blurring. I would, however, argue against allowing the traditional cues of our professional identity to erode.

Unlike most other businesses and professions, we physicians have a sacred contract with our patients. They allow us into the most private and intimate details of their lives. In return, we pledge to maintain stringent professional boundaries related to our behavior and give them the best of our intellect and compassion. Being addressed as "Doctor" is a constant reminder to me—and to everyone I interact with—of the oath I took to fulfill that pledge.

Please hold me accountable—and keep calling me "Doctor."

White Coats

After the (greatly appreciated!) multiple responses to my last entry on the "Doctor" title, I thought I'd expand the conversation to include another of those doctor identifiers: the white coat.

In my time in the medical world, I have seen a wide variety of attitudes from my medical colleagues regarding the white coat. Some appreciate the pockets. Some worry that the white coat may be off-putting to patients, especially disadvantaged ones. Some feel that it's an important symbol of the doctor-patient boundary. Some don't like having their style cramped by white polyester.

We physicians might make assumptions about what patients want us to look like, but what does the evidence say?

A cross-sectional survey in Tennessee a few years ago found that patients prefer family physicians who wear white coats.[1] Another study in a South Carolina internal medicine office found that patients "overwhelmingly" preferred physicians in white coats.[2] A Northeast Ohio OB residency found similarly; patients preferred a white coat and professional dress to scrubs.[3] A quick PubMed search pulls up the same theme over and over: the patients studied have more trust in and comfort with physicians who wear white coats.

We can misuse boundaries and labels, and they can chafe at times. But the chaos of a totally boundary-less world is equally unappealing. Patients already struggle at times to identify what role each of the people they interact with plays. In our hospital, the nursing students wear long white coats while physicians often favor fuzzy half-zip sweatshirts over their scrubs.

Some may argue that the above studies are not generalizable to the populations they care for. Others may describe their excellent patient relationships despite abolishing the white coat long ago. I'm certainly not discounting any of those thoughts; actually, I was quite surprised that my literature findings were so one-sided. I have to wonder if these studies are demonstrating our patients' desire to clearly identify who we are and, by extension, what we have pledged regarding our duty to them.

Fuzzy half-zip, I'll see you after work.

Notes

1. Amy J. Keenum, Lorraine S. Wallace, And Amy R. Barger Stevens, "Patients' Attitudes Regarding Physical Characteristics Of Family Practice Physicians," *Southern Medical Journal* 96, No. 12 (2004): 1190–94.

2. Shaikab U. Rehman Et Al., "What To Wear Today? Effect Of Doctor's Attire On The Trust And Confidence Of Patients," *The American Journal Of Medicine* 118, No. 11 (2005): 1279–86.

3. Ann Cha Et Al., "Resident Physician Attire: Does It Make A Difference To Our Patients?" *American Journal Of Obstetrics And Gynecology* 190, NO 5 (2004):1484–88.

Thursday, March 3, 2011

Googling "Family Medicine": Who's Defining Us?

After my last post, I started to wonder about my non-family-doctor readers. What if they are part of that large majority of people who really don't know what our specialty is all about? Where might they go to learn more about us?

Google, of course.

So here are the top three Google hits for "family medicine":

#1. Home page for the American Academy of Family Physicians: The AAFP's home page, not necessarily inappropriately, focuses on CME (continuing medical education) for members, advocacy, and public health issues. Some clicking around eventually leads to a "About the Specialty" page, which has lots more links. Click on one of them, scroll to the bottom of the page, and you'll find this: "Family medicine is the medical specialty which provides continuing, comprehensive health care for the individual and family. It is a specialty in breadth that integrates the biological, clinical and behavioral sciences. The scope of family medicine encompasses all ages, both sexes, each organ system and every disease entity."[1]

Hmmm. Maybe a little obtuse . . . if you manage to even find it buried in the site. Let's move on.

#2.   Family Medicine Journal, the official journal of the Society of Teachers of Family Medicine: As an STFM member, I receive and read this journal regularly. Much clicking around this site gives no succinct definition of family medicine. Again, not totally unreasonable given the site's focus.

#3.   Wikipedia. (C'mon, you knew it was coming.): "Family physicians deliver a range of acute, chronic and preventive medical care services. In addition to diagnosing and treating illness, they also provide preventive care, including routine checkups, health-risk assessments, immunization and screening tests, and personalized counseling on maintaining a healthy lifestyle. Family physicians also manage chronic illness, often coordinating care provided by other subspecialists. Many American family physicians deliver babies and provide prenatal care."[2]

I must admit—decently done, Wikipedia.

The Google hits further down start focusing on "find a local family medicine doctor" and family medicine residency programs. So truly, those people seeking to find a succinct answer about what our specialty is will probably stop with that Wikipedia link.

• • •

Dear National Family Medicine Organizations,

As a member of all of you, I implore you to add some simple definition of Family Medicine to your home pages. I get that promoting Family Medicine to the lay public isn't your main agenda for these sites, which are designed for physicians. (Though maybe it should be on the agenda somewhere.) But these sites are at the top of the Google "hit list" for our specialty, which confers responsibility on you. Don't make people dig through your sites to find out who we are, and don't leave the job of defining us to unsanctioned voices on Wikipedia.

We, as a specialty, must speak with a bolder and clearer voice.

Notes

1. American Academy of Family Physicians, "Family Medicine, Definition Of," accessed October 24, 2015, http://www.aafp.org/online/en/home/policy/policies/f/fammeddef.html.

2. Wikipedia, "Family Medicine," accessed October 24, 2015, http://en.wikipedia.org/wiki/Family_medicine/

The Same Look

It's been a hectic few weeks, with no time to even think about blogging. But, we've closed on our new house, I'm finally transitioning over work projects here, and the Singing Pen is glad to be back at the keyboard.

I spent most of my free time last week addressing letters to my patients that announce my out-of-state move and imminent departure. I handwrote every name in the "Dear" line and signed each one individually, so it took a while. I recognize that I performed this act entirely for myself; it was my opportunity to pause and reflect, if even for just a moment, about my relationship with each patient and family.

But the letters are starting to arrive at homes, and my patients are starting to arrive for their final appointments to say goodbye. I care for a diverse group: poor urban dwellers and university professors, young transplants to the area and four-generation families, white and African American and Iraqi and Vietnamese. Yet, despite their many differences, all my patients wear the same expression when our eyes first meet for these appointments.

Their chin points toward the ground, slightly, and their eyes look up at me, daring me to confirm the letter's truth. Accusations of abandonment are clearly evident in their wrinkled forehead, and their downturned lower lip hints at the sadness of a severed bond. The slight pinch of their nose displays unease, perhaps, with the unknown regarding their next doctor. They offer no words to me, waiting instead for me to speak first.

"So you got my letter," I usually say. I reassure them about their new family doctor here and share my joy in our relationship

155

and sadness in leaving. They wish me well and thank me for my care over the years. On and on these encounters repeat themselves, hour after hour and day after day. I accept this process as a necessary component of my departure.

But every one rips another small piece out of my heart.

It's About the Run

I remember well my final run at my favorite park in our old city just three weeks ago. The air was warm and the trees were rustling in the breeze as I jogged my well-loved loop. I didn't want to have to leave that park for the final time. Would I find in my new city someplace to run that was as Zen-inducing as that leafy, peaceful park?

I knew that it was time to move on, but I didn't want to leave my familiar job either. As much as I could intellectualize about the worthy reasons to go, some tenacious part of me balked at having to start over. What kind of a doctor would I be in a new place? Maybe I relied too much on the systems and people around me. Maybe getting plopped into a new spot would reveal my inadequacies. After all, I had spent the entire eight years of my post–medical school career in one place.

Leave we did, though, and here I am in my new job. Everything is unfamiliar, and I am humbled by having to relearn workflows and cultures. I still get lost in this office and our hospital across the street, though I certainly appreciate the gracious ways my new coworkers are assisting me.

My skills and experience are taking on new meaning here, and I'm coming to realize that my identity and purpose weren't as tied to my former office and program as I had feared. I brought my knowledge and personality with me, after all.

Last week, I pulled my running shoes out of a moving box and headed out into our new neighborhood for a jog. The neat sidewalks and flat topography are definitely different from my old city's feel, but as I trundled down the streets my feet moved just as they always had. The sky was wide and flat before me, clouds lazily ambling along. Children were playing in driveways surrounded by trees bursting with a million different shades of orange, red, and yellow. After the run, I experienced the same gentle burst of euphoria that I've always had.

I'm relieved to discover that I am more than the place that I left. My skills belong to me, regardless of the context I'm in. My enjoyment from running wasn't ultimately about the park, it was about the run itself. My job satisfaction wasn't ultimately about the place, it was about the work I was doing.

No matter where I go, I'm still a family doc.

My BHAG for Family Medicine

I have a BHAG (Big Hairy Audacious Goal).

I want people to hear "Family Medicine" and know that it refers to a medical specialty dedicated to providing relationship-based, patient-centered health care. I want people to know that family docs take care of a lot of complicated, challenging diseases—and not usually in isolation. Our patients have high blood pressure, complications from type 2 diabetes, congestive heart failure, depression, chronic kidney disease, emphysema, anxiety, asthma, and coronary artery disease—among others—and treating each such condition individually is nothing like treating two or more of them in relation to each other.

I want people to know that I trained for three years to become an expert in my specialty. During my Family Medicine residency, I learned about providing preventive care. I learned how to treat a multitude of acute problems—colds, fractures, lacerations, rashes, etc. I learned how to deliver babies, resuscitate victims of cardiac arrest, and drop a central line into a coding patient. I can take off your moles, skin tags, and warts. I can remove your ingrown toenail and treat your acne. I can obtain your pap smear, discuss your birth control options, and treat your STDs.

I want people to know that I can care for your kid and your grandparent. I routinely counsel teens about sex, drugs, and rock 'n' roll. I am comfortable in offices, hospitals, maternity wards, newborn nurseries, intensive care units, nursing homes, and even patients' homes.

I want people to know that Family Medicine residents learn about using the best medical evidence and the latest medical technology to guide decision-making conversations with patients. We residents can intelligently sift through the tremendous reams of medical studies that are published daily to pull out the information most relevant to their patients.

I want people to know that we residents learn how to work within a healthcare team. Nurses, medical assistants, pharmacists, care managers, social workers, administrative staff—it takes all of us to provide outstanding care. These incredibly important people are my hands, eyes, and ears when we take on the thousands of little tasks that must get done every day in the office and at the hospital.

I want people to know that no medical specialty is as devoted to medical education as Family Medicine. The Society of Teachers of Family Medicine holds an annual meeting devoted solely to medical student education. We are one of only a handful of medical specialties with an entire fellowship (i.e., post-residency training) devoted to faculty development—training the next generation of academic Family Medicine teachers, researchers, and leaders.

Lastly, I want people to know that we family docs do everything that we do in the context of our patients' belief systems, families, and communities. Our specialty is the only one that mandates dozens of hours of educational time during residency about the doctor-patient relationship. How to help folks quit smoking/overeating/whatever, how to tell someone that the biopsy did show cancer, how to mediate family disagreements about end-of-life wishes—these different types of behavioral instruction are just as important to a Family Medicine resident as the pathophysiology, treatment, and prevention of disease.*

If you're not a family doc, I bet you didn't know all of those things—and the blame for that truth lies squarely with us family docs. Frankly, other specialties have been better than us at promoting themselves. You all likely know what a dermatologist

160

or a cardiologist is, even if you're not working in the medical field. Family docs can learn a lot from how other specialties have advanced the interests of their patients by advancing their specialty's cause; it's something we have failed to recognize the importance of until now.

Because of that failure, Family Medicine is not understood—and thus not valued—by the public, by politicians, by health plan administrators, and by too many of the other people who make decisions about health care in this country.

We need to show them what Family Medicine is all about.

My BHAG is to share Family Medicine with the people who don't know about us yet. I hope that this blog does that in some small way; certainly, many of the Family Medicine bloggers and tweeters out there are doing it in a bigger way.

But I don't think that's enough. We need more. We need an #FMRevolution. I have to believe that there's something even bigger, hairier, and more audacious that we could do. I wish that I knew just what that that big, hairy, audacious thing was. Fortunately, though, I am but one of many.

It will take all of us to get the chorus of Family Medicine to echo across our nation.

---

* Am I saying that other specialties don't care about relationships with patients, patient-centered care, or evidence-based medicine? Absolutely not. But the statements above are true: other specialties do not systematically devote protected time in residency training about these issues the way Family Med residencies do. You could argue that other specialties don't need this training as much as family docs do, I suppose. But that's for a future post ... this post is about trying to boldly define our identity as a specialty. Lambasting other specialties is not on my agenda. Advancing the cause of Family Medicine is.

The Stack

Medical folk, you know what I'm referring to: that ever-
growing stack of journals that we'll all sit down and carefully
read through "someday."

My stack of journals is about three inches high at this
point. When I am in the groove of efficiency, I take the time to flip
through each journal when it arrives, tear out any articles that
look interesting, and recycle the rest. When the deluge of patient
care and teaching and research and meetings overtakes me, the
journals pile up unopened.

The Stack taunts me for my negligence. The Stack generates
guilt. The Stack hisses, "You can't keep up, you'll never keep up."

The Stack is right. I can't keep up. None of us can. The
medical literature machine cranks out hundreds of articles a
week. I do not have the hundreds of hours it would take to read
even a fraction of them. Accepting those facts is part of being
a twenty-first century physician. I don't want to abandon my
effort to stay up-to-date with the literature, but I need a new
strategy. Piles of journals that only accumulate dust aren't helping anyone.

I don't mean to suggest that journals are unnecessary—far
from it. I just need a different way to digest them. I do a decent
job of keeping up with Twitter, RSS feeds, and e-mail "breaking
news" alerts. I also use DynaMed and other evidence-based tools
on a daily basis.

While I respect those who like reading a paper journal, this
electronic effort is working much better for me. I'm usually one
of the first of my colleagues to know about a new study or a prac-

tice change recommendation, and I'm adept at quickly answering point-of-care questions using my electronic tools.

So, I'm done. Off go those unread journals to the recycle bin, and back I go to iGoogle, Twitter, InfoPOEMs, and the blogosphere.

I hereby declare myself free from The Stack.

Burnout & Redemption

I didn't consciously decide to put my blog on hiatus these last few months. I just got too busy one week to post, and then the next week, and then the next.

I admit to getting overwhelmed with some professional and personal challenges during this time. Part of my unintentional blog hiatus was certainly related to those issues; they were the only things I could think about, yet I didn't want to share them on this blog. The only problem was that those challenging situations were what I needed to write about.

The professional stuff, well, just isn't appropriate to share in a public space. And as for the personal stuff, I wish that I had the courage to share the details of my life with you all, but I don't. I love reading the medical bloggers who are bold enough to let us peer into their lives, and I'm grateful for their courage. Through their stories, we gain a deeper appreciation of our humanity. Blogging about the specifics of my personal issues, however, is just not for me. I'll reassure you that my health and marriage are fine, and that will have to sate whatever curiosity you might have. :)

As I look back on those four months, though, I recognize that more was going on than just challenging situations. I became emotionally overloaded. The trivial annoyances of my job became herculean, and I struggled to find the joy in being a doctor. It took more and more emotional energy every day to rally a positive facade with my patient care and teaching. I felt like I was stuck in an impossibly deep rut. I was burnt out. Would I ever love my job again?

Well, here's some advice adapted from a list that was published in JAMA:[1]

Strategies to Prevent Physician Burnout

Personal

Influence happiness through personal values and choices
Spend time with family and friends
Engage in religious or spiritual activity
Practice self-care (nutrition, exercise)
Adopt a healthy philosophical outlook
Have a supportive spouse or partner

Work

Gain control over one's environment and workload
Find meaning in work and set limits
Find a mentor
Have adequate administrative support systems

Easy, right? (Insert sarcasm here.) These goals are great for thinking about the long term and the big picture, but what about for when you're stuck in that rut? How do you clamber out?

I can only speak for myself, but I was pulled out of my rut this past weekend at the Family Medicine Education Consortium annual conference. 700+ family docs—and future family docs!—provided a whole lot of positive energy around our collective efforts to improve health for our patients and communities. They reminded me about why I felt called to this profession in the first place: I get to combine my science geek–ness with my drive to contribute to making the lives of those around me better. I get to interact with amazing people who inspire me to push the envelope even farther. I get the joy of being a "friend with special knowledge"[3] to my patients, and I get to contribute to the education of future family physicians, ensuring that they will deliver quality health care to generations to come.

For the long term, the strategies listed above are worth championing, but for the short term, try some time away from the office with your tribe.

Good-bye, rut. I'm back.

Notes

1. Anderson Spickard Jr, Steven G. Gabbe, and John F. Christensen, "Mid-Career Burnout in Generalist and Specialist Physicians," *Journal of the American Medical Association* 288, no. 12 (2002): 1447–50. http://jama.jamanetwork.com/article.aspx?articleid=195312/

2. Linda Gunderson, "Physician Burnout," *Annals of Internal Medicine* 135, no. 2 (2001), 145–48, http://www.eric.vcu.edu/home/resources/pipc/Other/Clinical_Skills/Article_Physician_Burnout.pdf .

3. "What Do I Want in a Doctor?" *Letters of Note*, accessed October 24, 2015, http://www.lettersofnote.com/2012/09/what-do-i-want-in-doctor.html.

Tuesday, November 20, 2012

Recipe for a Vital Primary Care Workforce

Thanksgiving is just around the corner, and so it seems appropriate to share a recipe:

Recipe for a Vital Primary Care Workforce

1. *Accept into medical school more students who are likely to choose a career in primary care.*

2. *Validate medical students' interest in primary care.*

3. *Provide adequate Family Medicine and General Internal Medicine training opportunities.*

4. *Enact meaningful payment reform.*

Now, a subpar cook such as me needs more than just the basics to pull off such a complicated recipe. So here are the details:

1. *Accept into medical school more students who are likely to choose primary care.*

Studies show that medical students who choose primary care are more likely to do or have done all of the following:

✓ Live in a rural area and/or plan to return to work in a rural area[1]

✓ Live in a disadvantaged area and/or plan to work in a disadvantaged area[2]

- ✓ Grow up in a low or middle socioeconomic neighborhood[3]
- ✓ Plan a career in a non-research field[4]
- ✓ Believe primary care is important and plan to practice primary care[5]
- ✓ Be indifferent to earning a high income after residency[6]
- ✓ Be female, older, and/or married[7]

2. Validate medical students' interest in primary care.

It's not enough to accept the right students into medical school; schools must also support interest in primary care. Here's what's been proven to increase the number of grads choosing primary care careers:

- ✓ Increasing mandatory rotation time in Family Medicine and General Internal Medicine[8]
- ✓ Rotating at two or more Family Medicine sites[9]
- ✓ Requiring a longitudinal primary care experience[10]
- ✓ Exposing students regularly to academically credible FM/GIM faculty[11]

3. Provide adequate Family Medicine and General Internal Medicine training opportunities.

Medical school graduate numbers are increasing as new schools open and existing schools expand their class size, but there are not enough residency slots for all of them. Some estimate that we will need 52,000 new primary care doctors by 2025, largely thanks to the Affordable Care Act,[12] and our capacity to train them is lacking. Additionally, few Internal Medicine residency graduates are practicing primary care these days, so the bulk of those 52,000 new primary care doctors will likely need to be Family Medicine docs. Unfortunately, Family Medicine residencies are not growing in numbers and capacity but are instead closing at an alarming rate.[13]

One of the local health systems here closed a Family Medicine residency program to "rebalance" their budget and workforce needs. Those GME [graduate medical education] slots are going to a vascular surgery residency. Local pressures are leading health systems to make short-sighted choices about what kind of medical specialties we are training our future physician workforce for.

4. *Enact meaningful payment reform.*

Payors devalue primary care by paying more for procedures and specialist care than for comprehensive, preventive primary care. Case in point: Our residency program practice earns about twice as much for doing a circumcision (a simple procedure that takes about ten minutes) than for admitting to the hospital a patient with complicated problems. We earn more for snipping off a skin tag than for providing forty-five minutes of direct patient counseling about chronic disease.

The current "Medicare physician payment formula . . . rewards volume over quality, and that discourages growth of primary care."[14] Systems produce what they are designed to produce, and right now our payment system disincentivizes primary care by better rewarding procedures and specialists. Unnecessarily expensive care does not produce better patient outcomes, and it certainly won't help the United States balance its bloated budget.[15]

Shifting our nation's health emphasis back to quality primary care will take deliberate effort by many parties. I would argue, however, that the payoff will be more than worth it. US counties with more primary care docs have lower health costs and longer life expectancies compared to counties with a heavier emphasis on specialists.[16] Yes, we need our specialist colleagues—but I'd argue that at this point in US history, we need Family Medicine more.

Notes

1. W. J. Kassler, S. A. Wartman, and Rebecca A. Silliman, "Why Medical Students Choose Primary Care Careers," *Academic Medicine* 66, no. 1 (1991): 41–43, http://www.ncbi.nlm.nih.gov/pubmed/1985676/

2. Janet H. Senf, Doug Campos-Outcalt, and Randa Kutob, "Factors Related to the Choice of Family Medicine as a Career," *Journal of the American Board of Family Practice* 16, no. 6 (2003): 502–12, http://www.ncbi.nlm.nih.gov/pubmed/14963077/

3. Kassler, Wartman, and Silliman, "Why Medical Students Choose Primary Care Careers"; Senf, Campos-Outcalt, and Kutob, "Factors Related to the Choice of Family Medicine as a Career."

4. Kassler, Wartman, and Silliman, "Why Medical Students Choose Primary Care Careers."

5. Kassler, Wartman, and Silliman, "Why Medical Students Choose Primary Care Careers."; Doug Campos-Outcalt, Janet H. Senf, and Randa Kutob, "A Comparison of Primary Care Graduates from Schools with Increasing Production of Family Physicians to Those from Schools with Decreasing Production," *Family Medicine* 36, no. 4 (2004): 260–64, http://www.ncbi.nlm.nih.gov/pubmed/15057616/

6. Kassler, Wartman, and Silliman, "Why Medical Students Choose Primary Care Careers."

7. C. J. Bland, L. N. Meurer, and G. Maldonado, "Determinants of Primary Care Specialty Choice: A Non-Statistical Meta-Analysis of the Literature," Academic Medicine 70, no. 7 (1995): 620–41, http://www.ncbi.nlm.nih.gov/pubmed/7612128/

8. Senf, Campos-Outcalt, and Kutob, "Factors Related to the Choice of Family Medicine as a Career."

9. Campos-Outcalt, Senf, and Kutob, "A Comparison of Primary Care Graduates from Schools with Increasing Production of Family Physicians to Those from Schools with Decreasing Production."

10. Bland, Meurer, and Maldonado, "Determinants of Primary Care Specialty Choice: A Non-Statistical Meta-Analysis of the Literature."

11. Bland, Meurer, and Maldonado, "Determinants of Primary Care Specialty Choice: A Non-Statistical Meta-Analysis of the Literature."

12. "Wanted: 52,000 More Primary Care Doctors by 2025," *The Fiscal Times*, November 19, 2012, http://www.thefiscaltimes. com/Articles/2012/11/19/Wanted-52000-More-Primary-Doctors-by-2025.aspx#page1/

13. http://www.ncbi.nlm.nih.gov/pubmed/14603401, http://www.ncbi.nlm.nih.gov/pubmed/1544533/, accessed November 2012 (site discontinued).

14. http://www.aafp.org/online/en/home/publications/news/news-now/government-medicine/20121107electionresults. html, http://www.hrsa.gov/advisorycommittees/bhpradvi sory/cogme/Reports/twentiethreport.pdf, accessed November 12 (site discontinued).

15. Guy Boulton, "Looming Primary Care Shortage Starts with Med School," *Milwaukee Wisconsin Journal Sentinel*, December 3, 2011, http://www.jsonline.com/business/looming-primary-care-shortage-starts-with-med-school-to-39lu9-134971463.html.

16. Barbara Starfield, "The Primary Solution: Put Doctors Where They Count," *Boston Review*, November 1, 2005, http://bostonreview.net/BR30.6/starfield.php.

Part 4
Discussions
Among the Writers

Introduction: Three Generations

By Beth Merenstein, PhD

Other than a small dip during the Great Depression in the 1930s, the number of physicians in the United States has steadily increased. But at same time, the number of family physicians has steadily declined.

The explanations for this are multifold. For one thing, family physicians tend to receive the lowest paychecks of all categories of physicians. Also, a lower level of prestige is sometimes associated with being a family physician. There is so much interest in this topic that journalist Karen Brown spent a year studying it, with the result being her documentary entitled *The Path to Primary Care: Who Will Be the Next Generation of Frontline Doctors?*

According to the Agency for Healthcare Research and Quality, in 2010, there were approximately 209,000 practicing primary care physicians in the United States. Of those, about 80,000 were practicing family physicians. According to the American Academy of Family Physicians, one in four office visits is made to a family doctor. As the number of family doctors declines, it becomes important to understand how family doctors see themselves. What role do they play, not only in the larger society but with regard to their patients and the system of health care? Furthermore, how do these interactions impact family doctors' understanding of themselves—of their very identity as doctors?

One way to begin to answer these questions is by looking at three individual family doctors from three different generations. By doing so, we can start to trace the relationships between generational differences, the trends these family physicians have experienced, and the larger social context in which they work. The three doctors in this worthwhile volume provide a fascinating look into the relationship between all three of these issues.

Looking at doctors from three different generations gives us many insights. First, by looking at the role of a family physician as he nears retirement, we can look back on a lifetime of patient-centered relationships. We can start to understand how a family doctor who began his career fifty years ago was centered in the world in a way very different from that of a physician entering medicine today.

Second, by listening to the words of a family doctor at his mid-career point, while recognizing that this means he entered the world of medicine about twenty-five years ago, we can think of the social issues evident in our society during the 1980s and 1990s.

And finally, hearing the concerns and considerations of a younger female family doctor, we can begin to understand what the world of medicine and the larger society is like in the 2000s. What matters here is not only when these doctors began their time practicing and what was happening in the larger social structure and culture but what that means in terms of their own identity as family doctors.

The Early Years of Family Medicine

Dr. Merenstein began his career as a family doctor at a time when there were few family physician practitioners. At the time, the more fragmented and specialized care that Americans received was viewed as a privilege that few could afford. The field of family medicine came about to challenge this notion, with its proponents arguing that family medicine could take care of the whole patient and his or her family. Arguing that medical care could and should be affordable, available, and accessible, these family doctors simultaneously expanded the role of medicine while making family practice a specialty.

Family medicine, like Dr. Merenstein, came of age as part of the Baby Boomer generation. At a time of great renewal and upheaval, this generation demanded expansion of every major societal institution. It pushed the boundaries of education, politics—and in this case, hospitals. The increasing demand to meet all the needs of this generation opened the door for an ever expanding family medicine specialty.

During this time, family medicine explored the idea of a more holistic approach to medicine. Believing that the doctor-patient relationship didn't need to center only on the doctor's office, family doctors of this time continued to engage in home visits. Though making house calls is clearly a practice that has fallen by the wayside, it remains one about which both doctor and patient continue to reminisce—as Dr. Merenstein describes in "The Doctor-Patient Relationship I," when he says, "We talked about the home visits I made when the girls were younger and we were all just starting out."

The structure of families in the United States underwent drastic changes during this time period. Divorce rates skyrocketed and then plateaued. Unprecedented numbers of women entered the workforce. Families had fewer children and waited longer to have those children. Whereas in the earlier part of the twentieth century, families stayed close together, as the decades moved on, adult children moved on as well—going where the jobs were. Cities and suburbs expanded at an ever increasing rate, and the institution of religion played a decreasing role in people's lives.

As Dr. Merenstein showcases here, he often helped families not only with their medical crises but also in dealing with changes and adjustments to the family structure. In "The Doctor-Patient Relationship III," he writes, "We spoke of various family difficulties, deaths of neighbors, conflicts with her son, and the financial problems. She noted repeatedly how dependent she was on her husband and how good he was to her and her children." Dr. Merenstein was practicing in a time of ever changing family, work, and geographic arrangements.

Placed within this context, the role of the family doctor had to adjust alongside the ever changing role of the family. Now there was even more of a need for a holistic doctor, one who would care for the totality of the patient and the patient's family. As the family physician, Dr. Merenstein played an ever important role in the lives of his patients.

In the first part of the twentieth century, communities were largely structured around farming, mining, and manufacturing economies. As a result, family medicine structured itself to meet the needs of people working in those communities. The community family doctor could and often would play the part of family negotiator, confidante, and therapist. As times changed and our society became structured more around a service economy in a more urban environment, the ways in which a family doctor supported the community changed as well. Dr. Merenstein saw these changes firsthand: he began practice in a more rural, mining community, working with a family practitioner with deep ties to the community—and then he saw the mines close down and the city encroach upon the rural community.

Practicing in smaller, more intimate communities can more easily bring out the holistic role of the family doctor, as Dr. Merenstein suggests in his piece "The Family Doctor—A Tribute." As he says of his original partner at his rural practice: "He delivered most of the young people in both communities and was the only doctor for those communities and the multiple small suburban areas that defined the 1950s. Some forty years later, I am trying to involve our residents with the urban neighborhoods we serve in a way that was natural to Dr. Waite."

This approach to family medicine during this time offered something unique that in many ways cannot be replicated in our current times. As Dr. Merenstein explained about both Dr. Waite, and himself:

Of course, he saw more patients in their homes than in his own. We made regular home visits each day between morning and afternoon hours. The only indication was that someone wanted one. You don't need to take much of a social history when you live with people and visit the sick in their homes. It's possible on those home visits to diagnose acute cholecystitis with an unusual presentation when you recall the patient's mother and grandmother presented the same way. Cost-effective analysis isn't needed either. When you make daily house calls, you say to those who can't afford to pay, "The man's sick and needs to be seen. Don't worry about paying for it.

This method worked during a time of limited communications technology and significantly limited managed care. But we see, as the years went on, that Dr. Merenstein's colleagues felt pulled in different directions.

Throughout his career, Dr. Merenstein reflected his generation's ideologies, perspectives, and moral compass. The patient's concerns and decision making were part of the process, patients were treated in a holistic way, family needs and expectations were also important pieces of the patient improvement process, and there was a persistent recognition that not everyone could be—or should be—mended completely. When Dr. Merenstein retired, he acknowledged that he was as worried about leaving medicine as his patients were about his leaving. He details this in "What Will I Do Without You?" He writes, "The patient-physician relationship has sustained me and my patients and I hope contributed to our health and quality of life."

The Mid-Career Years

Our mid-career family doctor, Dr. Han, entered his professional career at a time of growth in the practice of family medicine. Not only was the number of medical schools increasing, but so too was the number of those entering family medicine as a specialty. Family medicine made inroads into academia and community clinics, and it established new residency programs. According to Robert B. Taylor, "The promise of family medicine was to return America's health care to a generalist-based model, led by family physicians who could provide quality health care for 80 to 90 percent of the health care needs of their patients."[1]

Furthermore, Dr. Han was part of a larger social demographic change. As the post-1965 Immigration Laws opened up our society to vast new populations, largely from Asian and Latin American countries, our country's diversity took on new dimensions. Where previously we had existed along a largely white-black racial divide, now we were entering a world more nuanced and varied in terms of race and ethnicity. As a Korean American, Dr. Han understood these changes personally and professionally. As he explains in "The Kindest Insult," patients often expected things of him he felt he could not provide: "What was painfully upsetting to me, however, was the anger and offence she took at my need for a Korean language interpreter."

After trying unsuccessfully to connect to his Korean patient, Dr. Han finally mutters one of the few words he remembers in Korean from childhood, and in doing so, totally alters his relationship with his patient. "I never asked her why she suddenly accepted my cultural naïveté, or what motivated her to tolerate my inadvertent affront to Korean pride that was inherent in my inability to be a 'native speaker.' Perhaps my remark was the kindest insult she had ever received, which had arisen out of my desperation as a fellow Korean who, like her, was in many ways still a foreigner in America."

Yet while he might have been able to connect to his Korean and other Asian patients, Dr. Han also experienced what many others of this generation were forced to face: a lingering prejudice and discrimination. In particular, Asians and Asian-Americans in the 1970s and 1980s were often subject to fierce forms of racism, with lingering and misplaced resentment stemming from the Vietnam and Korean wars. As Dr. Han recollects in "Welcome to the Arctic Circle," "I grew up experiencing much racism and prejudice. Facing provocative racist taunts by children and adults alike and being ridiculed for my Asian features were painful reminders of my 'perpetual foreigner' status....Feeling somewhat lost, somewhere in between cultures of Korea and America, I searched for a place to fit in, to be anonymous, to not stand out simply because of my physical appearance. These struggles of identity intensified as I grew older, even as I moved toward a career in medicine."

During this time (the 1990s), medicine was seen as more of a generalist practice, with the majority of physicians seeking this type of practice. Additionally, managed care was the new direction of the health care structure, with a focus and an emphasis on cost-efficient practices. Ironically, this was also a time of increased prosperity for those in the upper echelons of society. Because of this, we began to see even more inequality arise between those who could afford care and those who could not. As health management organizations (HMOs) proliferated, doctors were under pressure to minimize costs, reduce time spent with patients, and pull back on any "extras" such as home visits.

As George Ritzer explains in his book *The McDonaldization of Society*, American society during this time period saw the widespread application of four particular principles: efficiency, calculability, predictability, and control. Though modeled on the McDonald's franchise, these principles were successfully applied to many of our core institutions, including the world of medicine. As Ritzer argues, "Doc-in-a-box can also be more efficient than private doctors' offices because they are not structured to permit the kind of personal (and therefore inefficient) attention patients expect from their private physicians."[2]

As we can surmise from the writings of Dr. Han, he began his career in this "McDonaldized" culture and structure, going into family medicine to help the totality of the patient yet increasingly being forced to pull back from this ability and desire. Through his years of patient care, he witnessed the increasing economic divide—the widening gulf between the affluent and the fully insured and between the poorer and the federally insured—and he was forced to acknowledge the difference in care these patients received. In "Malignant Neglect," when he asked a resident examining a woman presenting long-term pain and discomfort why her adrenal disease went untreated for so long, the resident simply replied, "'Lack of medical insurance,' without missing a beat."

As more and more Americans came to depend on an employer-based health care structure, family doctors witnessed the too real consequences of this system. As Dr. Han also writes in "Malignant Neglect":

The final obstacles that prevented Mrs. Waite from getting medical care were her lack of health insurance and the scarcity of clinicians for the uninsured. The Waites lived in a town located within a federally designated medically underserved area. Only one sporadically staffed "free clinic" and one family-planning clinic were available to provide care to uninsured patients, and the Waites were unaware of these resources. To make matters worse, even if Mrs. Waite had qualified for Medicaid, many local clinicians did not accept Medicaid patients because of low reimbursement, so outpatient health care would have been just as inaccessible to her.

Ironically, it was during the managed care era of the 1980s and 1990s that the public began to recognize that much of the population was underserved by the health care system. The uninsured and underinsured population was skyrocketing during this time; by the late 1990s and early 2000s, approximately 45 million Americans fell into one of those two categories. Family doctors like Dr. Han wanted to treat all patients yet were forced to recognize that policies in place often wouldn't let them do that. For example, in his story "Serious Side Effects," Dr. Han relates the case of one such patient: "Then his health insurance premiums rose to unaffordable heights—and, three months into his cancer treatment, he'd lost his insurance coverage. Unable to afford care on his own, he'd stopped being treated."

Additionally, Dr. Han was pushed to spend less time with patients, see more patients, and move away from those patients who couldn't afford more costly medical care. Working within this context, Dr. Han and his fellow family physicians worked hard to alleviate the struggles of those patients. Their efforts were not unique, as rising health care costs, increased control by large HMOs, and health insurance in an employer-based structure required more ingenuity on the part of the family doctors on the front lines. The purpose of family medicine has always been patient centered with a holistic approach; yet, the changes to the insurance structure that developed in the 1990s through today have caused many family physicians to struggle to continue doing what they should do and want to do. As Dr. Han points out in "Serious Side Effects," at his family medicine–based medical center, "Taken as a whole, these patients represent every permutation of wealth and insurance status (including the complete lack of it). Compassionate, patient-centered medicine calls for physicians to respond empathically and care for every patient, validating each individual as unconditionally deserving of care."

During this time period of ever increasing health care costs and an ever more impersonal system, family doctors such as Dr. Han were forced to maneuver and consider issues in a far different manner from previous generations of physicians such as Dr. Merenstein. As Dr. Han says in "Passing the Torch," "Health care policymakers and administrators continue to move the responsibility for increasing costs onto the physicians and hospitals themselves, implicitly placing the 'blame' for illness and bad outcomes on physicians."

The Younger Generations

There are two key characteristics that make the younger generations of family doctors different from earlier generations: (1) a dependence on and expectation of technology, and (2) a recognition of the rise of women and minorities in the education and professional realms. This generation—loosely, the Millennium Generation—is the most media-connected cohort. Millennials spend more time watching television, listening to music, playing video games, and interacting with friends on computers. Distinctly different from the previous two generations, Millennials have grown to depend on computers and the Internet.

Although technically a Gen Xer, Dr. Jen Middleton's experiences as a family physician illustrate this new utilization of and dependence on technology. She writes a blog in which she addresses the various issues she comes across as a family doctor. Originally, she was reluctant to put her own thoughts out on the Web, but then she began to read Twitter and marveled at "the incredible depth of medical writing and thought generating that happen behind the scenes of those 140-character posts. The opportunity to advocate for family medicine and share my stories in this new format was too tempting to pass up, and The Singing Pen of Doctor Jen was born."

Dr. Jen's perspective allowed her to simultaneously recognize the potential for using technology in medical advancement and the older generation's resistance to it. As she writes in "A Paper Cut in a Digital World," "The majority of the attending staff, as you are probably already imaging, did not share my optimism. They were unhappy with the clunkiness I alluded to above. They didn't want to take the time to log in, pull up the right patient, open a new progress note, and type in their thoughts. 'Too many clicks' became their mantra."

This perspective also helped her recognize that since anything can be found online now, paper journals—though very useful fifty years ago—are no longer the only or even the most reliable source of medical information. As Dr. Middleton writes in "The Stack,"

"While I respect those who like reading a paper journal, this electronic effort is working much better for me. I'm usually one of the first of my colleagues to know about a new study or a practice change recommendation, and I'm adept at quickly answering point-of-care questions using my electronic tools. So, I'm done. Off go those unread journals to the recycle bin, and back I go to iGoogle, Twitter, InfoPOEMs, and the blogosphere."

This connection with and dependence on social media makes Millennials both potentially less socially adept and more globally aware than any previous generation. Their focus on technological advances can also lead them to an amplified interest in the role of their identity in the larger social context. Having a greater appreciation of the global environment can lead them to ask where they fit in, and it has caused Dr. Middleton to explore her experience of being a physician. Furthermore, family physicians' blogging and tweeting helps them create a social media community in which they can engage with their concerns, question their own legitimacy, and share uncertainties and affirmations.

The Millennial Generation's interest in and concern with the personal and individual allow them to engage in a more nuanced examination of not only those they treat but also their fellow physicians. One of Dr. Middleton's first pieces—"Today I'm Grieving a Physician Suicide"—suggests this ongoing concern. Whereas previous generations were more hesitant to openly discuss depression and mental illness, particularly among medical professionals, this generation is more willing to challenge the stigma attached to such illnesses. As Dr. Middleton expresses in her thoughts for her deceased friend and colleague, "I worry that this 'macho mentality' of medicine may have dissuaded you from confiding your suicidal thoughts to anyone."

The Millennium Generation is also a more individually focused and self-aware generation. They tend to be concerned with questions of identity and understanding one's place in the larger world, and they have a strong belief that agency can alter one's path in life. Millennial family physicians will therefore approach medicine this way, as Dr. Middleton explains in the same piece: "I do not think that my treatment goals themselves have changed, but I hope that my interactions with patients now express better the depths of my concern for them and my genuine desire to understand them as individuals."

Additionally, the Millennial Generation is the most racially and ethnically diverse. Due to a combination of higher birthrates among minority populations and an ever growing immigrant population, over 35 percent of this population are people of color. Members of this generation are also more likely to have grown up in nontraditional family units, with one in four having grown up in single-parent homes, and three out of four having grown up with working mothers.

On a related note, over 50 percent of new medical students are female, suggesting that females will represent the majority of all physicians within a generation. Within the health care fields, we see a distinction in the kind of medicine women are more likely to practice: of final-year residents within pediatrics, 73 percent are female; within family medicine, 55 percent are female; and within OB/GYN, 83 percent are female.[3]

This change has been noticed by patients as well, as Dr. Middleton writes in "Fallibility/Forgiveness": "It's so wonderful to see young women these days being doctors. In my day, we had to settle for being nurses. Not that nursing isn't noble, mind you. But it was our only choice."

Women in our society are socialized to be caring, nurturing, and more emotionally competent than men. As more women enter the field of medicine, it's possible to see some of these characteristics entering into the professional world of medicine as well. As Dr. Middleton writes in "Our Family Doctor," as she worked with a family experiencing the impending loss of a loved one, she repeated the "mantra" she had heard an ICU nurse give to families so many times: "We'll give him a beautiful death." Going on to describe her own emotions, she says, " I remember wondering if real doctors were supposed to cry with their families." For Dr.

Middleton, having been socialized and mentored in a world of primarily male doctors, she wonders how much she is actually allowed to "care" and show emotion for her patients.

Dr. Middleton fits within the parameters of the Millennial Generation. In her stories, we first see her acknowledgement of the expanding role technology is coming to play in medicine. She does not rely solely on technology to take her place but sees the importance technological advancements can offer the current and future state of medicine. Further, she continuously asks questions about her role as a physician. She questions the place of family doctors and how her identity, both as a woman and a doctor, continue to be shaped by her place in the institution of medicine.

· · ·

All three of the physicians who wrote stories for this volume have created professional and personal practices based on understanding family medicine within the contexts and confines of their lives. They have seen changes in the practice of medicine, and most particularly in the development of family medicine. Within their own understandings and identities based on race/ethnicity, gender, and class, they have learned to negotiate what being a family doctor means at very different times in history. We can begin to see how their generational differences have affected not only their relationships with their patients, but their insights into themselves as doctors.

Notes

1. Robert B. Taylor, "The Promise of Family Medicine: History, Leadership, and the Age of Aquarius," *Journal of the American Board of Family Medicine* 19, no 2 (2006): 183–90.

2. George Ritzer, *The McDonaldization of Society* (Thousand Oaks, CA: Pine Forge Press, 2004), 52.

3. *AMA Physician Master File (2012).*

Why Do We Write?

In this section of the book, we—the three physician/authors —will share transcripts of conversations among us about our writing, including why we wanted to write this book. We'll also explore the commonalities and differences behind our approaches to writing and patient care as they relate to our different life stages and generations.

JOEL: One of the things I wanted to talk about is why we write these stories and why we decided to combine our writing into a book. I'm not sure why I do it, but the idea is that I'm sharing my experiences with other people and other physicians so that we can all learn from those experiences. Putting these ideas into a book has the potential to bring them to a wider readership.

I also think I write partially to see what people pick up from my stories. Others often see things in a person's writing that the writer himself didn't see. I know that editors have picked up a focus or idea in a story I wrote that I never thought of when I was writing it.

Another reason people write is just due to an urge to write and share their thoughts. I know that in practicing medicine, I would sometimes see a patient and make a note about him or her, knowing that some aspect of his or her situation would make a good story. But I had to keep reminding myself that storytelling was not the primary reason for me seeing patients. My job was to be their doctor first and to write the story later, making it secondary.

JON: I agree with Joel. I have always really enjoyed stories but never thought of writing them down. In family medicine, we pride ourselves in creating relationships and taking care of people. Most of the time when people are talking to us in the office, they're telling stories—intense stories—and we become part of the story. I realize that even as a teacher, I spent most of my time teaching by using stories rather than quoting a lot of literature; that was one of my most effective teaching methods and something I enjoyed doing. There was also the practical point of trying to write down stories because I enjoyed listening to them and I enjoyed telling them—so it was kind of fun to write them too.

JEN: I guess for me it's a little different. Writing down the things that happened to me was initially just journaling. I didn't write these stories intending to get them published and share them with people. They were just my deeply personal thoughts about experiences that profoundly affected me and that I needed to process. So for me, writing was a way to process both the beautiful and amazing things that happened to me as well as the very difficult experiences I've had.

It never occurred to me do anything with those journal entries until I got to know Joel and Jon and they introduced me to narrative writing in medicine. Some of these stories I felt compelled to share because they contained a message I felt strongly about. But I can't honestly say that I have ever sat down to write with a plan from the get-go to publish. Most of the stuff I've written down I will never publish, which is OK with me.

JOEL: It's important to point out that this is not a new idea. Doctors have been writing stories for centuries. Probably the most famous doctor/storyteller in modern times was William Carlos Williams, who started out not being sure if he wanted to be a doctor or a writer—and did both well. Rita Charon has in recent years revitalized the idea of the narrative in medicine and has been a leader in what is a resurgent movement in narrative medicine. She has even pushed the point that stories tell us the way we should practice medicine.

I was impressed to hear a talk by Robert Coles—a psychiatrist at Harvard who is probably retired now and a protégé of William Carlos Williams. Coles would meet a patient to take a history, and he would not say, "Tell me why you're here and what I can do for you." Instead, he would say, "Tell me your story." So I think what we're saying, in too many words, is that medicine is about telling stories, sharing stories, and using the story to help with diagnosis and treatment. But it's always a story, and we just try to repeat, record, and share it.

JON: I went to a poetry workshop this summer, and the poet who led it was an accomplished writer and teacher. She said some pretty encouraging things about writing. She said I was really lucky to be a physician who was interested in writing because in society, we physicians are still held with some degree of esteem and respect and people will actually listen to us if we write things that are interesting and provocative.

She's working on some poetry about the environment, and she made the point that it's important to have a voice and to speak from that voice about issues of social concern and social responsibility. Then she made a self-deprecating joke: "You know I'm a poet—it's what I do, and I would like my words and messages to get out—but many people won't read me because I'm 'just a poet.'"

I felt really sad to hear that because she's a wonderful poet and her words are remarkable. But she had a very practical point in what she was saying about encouraging physicians to write, especially about issues of social justice.

JEN: Jon, I think you're right and that poet was right that we physicians do have significant power, but I think the cool thing about most of the physicians' narrative writing that I see is that it's very humbling most of the time. We write about things that didn't go well or about our mistakes, for example. I think it's a nice way of equalizing the doctor and the patient at the end of the day. When we humble ourselves before our patients and our audience, it helps us remember our humanity. Physicians' narratives can show that, despite all the twenty-first century medical technologies, we still care at the end of the day about our patients' stories.

JOEL: Part of it is confusing to me, because patients have told me something different. *JAMA* [*Journal of the American Medical Association*] has narratives in the section called "A Piece of My Mind," which I think is one of the most universally read sections, and often the stories are about difficult doctor/patient relationships. Yet when you talk to patients, they say their doctor doesn't practice the way it's depicted in the story. If doctors love that way of practicing so much and read about it and identify with it, why don't they practice that way?

Maybe we do and we just don't appreciate it, but it seems to me that there's a need for patients to have these stories told and that they really like the idea of a physician sharing these stories. I'm just not sure why they aren't—or maybe they are, I just don't know—but why is that sentiment not more universal?

Did you want to add anything, Jon? As I said before, we may pick out some themes about why we write, but people who are reading this may have different ideas about what we're saying.

JON: One of things I was thinking, as Jen did a nice summary about the different themes, was talking about humility. Should we talk about why we are doing this book in particular first, before we talk about the themes?

JOEL: I think that's a good idea.

JEN: I think that's reasonable.

JON: Joel, I think you should talk about your ideas of writing about medicine across the generations and then talk about fallibility, as Jen suggested. That might be the bridge to talk about other themes.

JOEL: Let me think about it while I talk about it. I think that one of the things that is unique about our book is that we are of three different generations. I'm retired, Jon is in his prime, and Jen is early in her career. I guess some important questions from those three different perspectives are these: Do our stories have the same ring? Are we dealing with the same issues? We deal with the doctor-patient relationship, responsibility, death and dying, and the question "Who am I as a doctor versus who am I as a person?" But are there some different perspectives on those themes and topics that we have because we are in different stages of life?

I think it was Ralph Waldo Emerson who said, "You could say one thing today and really believe and say the opposite tomorrow." Maybe I'm remembering that because of the political atmosphere right now. So I might say something now that I might disagree with at another time.

Right now, I would say that despite the differences between our generations, despite our different examples, we're dealing with the very same issues in similar ways. I'm trying to figure out—even after forty-two years of practice—who I am as a doctor, what my responsibilities are, what my story brings to it, and what my story brings beyond making a diagnosis and writing a prescription. If there's a difference in perspective across generations, I think it's our job to identify that because I think that's one of the key aspects of this book we can emphasize.

Maybe the two of you can come up with some ideas and I can then think about it and come back. Do you think we have something to say that's different, looking at ourselves and our patients?

JEN: I feel our themes have more similarities than differences. Some of the mediums are different, like my blog, but I'm not sure if I can really find a lot of differences. We know things about medicine that are different now than they were forty years ago, but those things are not what the three of us are writing about. We're not writing about electronic health records and all the fancy radiographic tools that we have now. It doesn't seem to be the essence of what we're mostly writing about. At the end of the day, it is mostly about our patients and who they are—and that's unchanged to me.

JON: That is a good point, and maybe the reasons we write tell us more about ourselves as storytellers. It's interesting to look at us as writers across the generations. I got started kind of late writing. I think it's pretty cool, Jen, that you started and have been writing even while you were training, and you talked before about how you always enjoyed writing. I find it interesting reading about other writers who say they were born to write or couldn't stop writing—that it's such an integral part of them that they *had* to write, journal, and finally publish something. Since I've been writing for only the last ten years, I've been drawn to this idea of looking at this across generations, but what Jen said makes sense to me: there are a lot of similarities; we like to tell stories about how patients have affected us and what they've taught us too. So maybe the story for me is why I waited so long to start writing, or how Jen started so early, and how Joel has been writing throughout his long career. And Joel has been doing scientific writing too, which is very different.

JOEL: Even though I agree, I would like us to try and focus, because if we have a point about three generations, there must be some differences that we're not thinking of. Similarities are easier to identify. I'm interested in writing about saying good-bye to patients, but Jen has done that too. And Jon has moved a couple times, so you've had to think about the questions: where am I now, where am I going, and what is going on? I know that for me, part of it is about loss and absence. I wrote one story in which I asked, "What will I do without you?" I concluded that saying good-bye was going to be harder for me than my patients—and that has been true. In many ways I was more dependent on being part of that doctor-patient relationship than they were—or maybe I just thought more about it. I don't know. I don't think you're aware of it when you're right in the middle of it, and certainly not when you're beginning. It defines who you are and defines your concept. It might have been more of an issue for me in my generation than for either of you.

JEN: I don't know, Joel, I think a lot of what I've experienced since moving has been struggling with a new definition of myself. I had a brief period of time from my last day with all of you to the first day of my current job when I wasn't anyone's doctor—and that was very, very unsettling. I had come to a new place and had to start all over at square one with every single patient to build relationships.

I definitely was mourning the loss of the relationships I had built in my previous job. I had been with my patients for eight years in Pittsburgh before I left—and while that's not forty-two years, I saw babies I delivered go to elementary school, at least. I'm only just now starting to get to know my new patients here, only just starting to feel as if I have my feet underneath me again. If that happened to me after just eight years in a place, I can't imagine what it would be like after forty-plus years.

JOEL: One of the things you mentioned before, which a lot of people think about, is that medicine is practiced so differently now. Recently, there was an entire page in *The New York Times* devoted to the digitalization of medical care, and one of the reasons I retired is that I can't keep up with computers, digital equipment, and the new ways of practicing. I wonder if in your younger generations, that makes a difference in these stories. Are the stories different because of computers and the new diagnostic aids? Some people are saying that the stethoscope is going to disappear and new gadgets will be invented, and maybe medicine will be totally different—and you two are going through that transition. Is it very difficult to go through that transitional stage? It was easy for me to get out of it.

JON: That's an interesting point, because in the last twenty or so years, documenting patient care has changed dramatically. When I was a resident, we actually had two different charts: the original note would go into the hospital chart, with a photocopy of the notes you wrote for the family health center chart. You would have to finish all your notes and do all this crazy photocopying stuff. Now it's so automated, using the computer, but when we started using electronic health records eight years ago or so, it was difficult on so many levels trying to learn this technology because it was a skill we just had to learn on the fly.

I think all in all, despite my anger or resistance to change, I still had a pretty well-rounded sense of what being a doctor was, so I kind of knew what the means-versus-the- ends were. There are so many frustrations in dealing with managed-health companies and micromanagement by managed-care medical directors, and the paperwork burden has not decreased because of electronic health records. However, I will say that using electronic health records does streamline prescribing.

I still think the core of family medicine is there in day-to-day practice. My father has been very ill recently. I've gone with him to see some of his doctors, and I can tell you the specialists he has seen have been wonderful. But the way the specialists use a computer is so different from the way we do, and I think as family physicians we put some premium on how we communicate with people, and we try to be thoughtful about using the computer as the third presence in the room.

Seeing how specialists use the computer—basically doing hunt-and-peck on the computer keys, looking up at the patient occasionally, and making the patient sit through about half an hour of silence while trying to write their notes (out of a forty-minute consultation, maybe ten of those minutes was talking and another four or five examining the patient, while the rest of the time was watching the specialist type on a computer—left me more than a little bit frustrated. It made me appreciate what we do as family physicians because I think we are really invested in relationships because we want to help guide people, advise people, and be with them. It shows that we're very different from other specialists whose primary focus is on the disease process.

JOEL: I think as family physicians we need to do that, but we should expect the specialist to also be human. Have we really done the job in family medicine to say that we continue to hear the stories, and tell these stories, while the computer is there?

JON: Not yet; I think that process is still evolving. But I think we're at least looking at that as something that needs to be taught and developed, rather than focusing on the diagnostic technologies and the latest tests. The computer needs to be just another tool to help patients.

JEN: I agree. I think that family medicine, in many ways, has been a trailblazer with medical education. Family medicine invented the idea of a behavioral health curriculum and teaching doctor-patient communication skills, and our specialty was among the first to require every resident to have time dedicated to learning those skills. Similarly, as far as I know, ours is the only residency specialty that includes computer skills in its residency training. It's kind of cool that the same folks who prized the value of the story were the leaders in saying we have this new tool and that there may be changes, and also in asking how we should mitigate those changes and use computers to our advantage and our patient's advantage. We family doctors have been proactive about studying the things we do with computers and determining which of those things help our relationship with patients and which of them hurt.

JOEL: While I was precepting and things were changing—diagnostic tests, new treatments—I would say to the learner, student, or resident, "That is all good. But when you close the door and go in the room with the patient, it's the same as it's always been: it's just you and the patient." But that's not so anymore, because when you close the door, there are three of you: you, the patient, and the computer—and we really have to learn the best way to manage that. Do you think our stories help in any way, or do they have any message in terms of the new way of practicing with the computer? I have a friend who was close to ninety-five years old who said he retired because he couldn't pay attention to the patient's story since he had to be on the computer. That is not a fair trade-off as far as I'm concerned.

JON: Maybe by telling stories, we'll always come back to how we are with the patient herself, and it will just be a reminder that the primary focus of what we're supposed to be doing is taking care of our patients—and also ourselves, which many times we don't do a very good job of either. We've written about that topic too.

JOEL: Yes, we have.

JEN: I'm the poster child for that.

JOEL: We've all written about that.

JEN: That's true, Joel. I don't want to assume that I'm speaking for everyone in my generation, but I like the computer a lot, and I miss the computer now in a new job that still uses paper records. I felt I was able to give better care more efficiently with the computer. I could spend a couple more minutes talking to patients because of the things the electronic record helped me to do. I found it to be a positive change. In my prior practice, I had one or two patients who were really opposed to me using a computer, so I just didn't use it with them, but the rest of the patients were accepting.

You can do a lot of cool things with the computer screen, sharing information directly with the patient—"Look, here's junior's growth chart," or "Look, here's the trend of your A1c." You can use it to enhance the doctor-patient relationship, but I think you can only do that if you're being intentionally thoughtful about doing so. I'm trying to think if any of the narrative pieces I've read involved a computer. It's interesting to me that it's affecting us but we're not writing about it.

JOEL: John Frey, a family doctor in Wisconsin, wrote an essay in *JAMA* called "At a Loss for Words," about how he enjoyed making personal notes in the margins of his handwritten patient care notes but couldn't do that with a computer. I'm sure there's a way that people like you, Jen, can figure out how to do that even with a computer, but that's the only way to make more personal observations about a patient that I can think of. It was really interesting to me that you said that using the computer could give you more time with a patient. Soon after I was in medical school, over fifty years ago, Jack Myers was the chair of medicine at Pitt, and he was known as a supreme diagnostician, a man who knew everything. Jack got very into computers when they first came out, and he said the prime focus of the computer is to give the doctor more time to talk to the patient. I don't know that everybody believes that, but that was his goal and I think that should be a motivation for us.

JEN: If you're only using it as another way of documenting, it's not going to give you any more time because it takes just as long to type something in as it does to dictate. But if you're using it to automate things like refills, test ordering, getting results faster, and looking through charts, then I do think all of those things happen more quickly. All of those seconds are precious to me. Now that I'm back temporarily in a paper-based world, I want those seconds back that I have to spend doing all that stuff. It's aggravating.

JOEL: Maybe one of you can write a story emphasizing the human side of medicine together with the computer.

JEN: I'm completely uninspired to do that in the paper world I'm currently living in.

JOEL: You can't be inspired by it in advance—it has to come upon you while it's happening or after.

JON: I think the danger with electronic health records is the time incentive to truly depersonalize everybody and have every patient encounter fit into some prewritten format. A doctor in Chicago wrote a hilarious and compelling essay in *JAMA* titled "Copy and Paste." In it, the author wrote a story about a patient just repeating the same paragraphs of information over and over without meaning—because that's what people do in electronic health records, essentially turning every patient encounter into a repository of yes-or-no answers.

What we're supposed to do is go back to telling stories, but that's very difficult and I think a little more time consuming than the "usual" kind of patient interview: just asking questions to get yes-or-no answers and sticking the answers in a chart. People who are good at using the computer while still connecting to the patient—like you, Jen; or John Frey; or Jack Myers; who had the intention of using the computer to have more time with the patient —are very good at translating what the patient's story is, using the computer effectively as a means rather than an end in itself.

JOEL: How would you use the computer with the idea of saying to patients, "Tell me your story"?

JEN: When I was on computers at St. Margaret, I very rarely used the software program checkboxes to document the subjective story of the patient. I almost always free- texted the subjective into the note in an abbreviated format. I could not stand the little check-boxes. I tried using them a couple times—I wanted to be open to new ways of doing things—but I felt that particular software program, as you said, depersonalized the patients too much. I wanted to be able to look at a patient's notes and see the patient's story.

However, the checkboxes for the patient physical exam are a total timesaver—I love it. You have no idea how many times a day I dictate virtually the same physical exam on somebody who is relatively normal. Now I have to write down that I'm ordering an X-ray and dictate that I ordered it. With the EHR [Electronic Health Record], I can put that in one place and have it document-ed that I ordered it—it's in my notes, done. The history of present illness and also the assessment (which I still free-text) are entered in my Epic notes. I'm a fast typist from years of writing, and I was able to integrate that pretty seamlessly after a few awkward starts with my patients.

JOEL: Every patient, every visit should start with a brief story and then go to the checklist. But first is the story, because there *is* a story. I hate to go this far back, but Hippocrates says it is often more important what person has the disease than what disease the person has, and I think that's the kind of thing that comes out in a story—which doesn't come out when you just check boxes in a computer program.

JEN: I think that's true.

JOEL: So maybe we can talk a little bit more specifically about what we have in this book. Jon, will you start with a favorite story of your own that you want to say something about—to see if we get any response from readers or listeners as to whether they find something in your story that you didn't find?

JON: Going back to how and why we write and our personal evolution, the first piece I ever wrote, "Welcome to the Arctic Circle," came out of a writing workshop led by Paul Gross in Cleveland at Northeast Society of Teachers of Family Medicine. I walked into the meeting thinking the topic of narrative medicine was interesting. During the writing exercise portion of the seminar, I wrote this piece very quickly.

The opening lines of this story were really great. I was working in rural Alaska years ago, and I met this woman in the emergency room—and the first thing she said to me was "You're a f–ing Korean." Writing that story in that workshop was so liberating! Of course, it was not so liberating when she said it to me in person, but actually it was kind of humorous.

So I wrote the story, fleshed it out, and had it published. And then I realized that there were so many stories like that—stories about racism and injustice that also had a tinge of humor, which is one of the best ways to deal with difficult issues like that. I felt that writing this story was really a powerful way to not forget and to maybe teach something through a story. So I guess that goes back to why we're family physicians and why we've chosen a path in terms of teaching.

JEN: I'm trying to think of a theme for mine. I guess for me, all of the things I wrote were intensely personal. I have put all of my efforts into blogging the last couple of years, and I haven't worked to get a narrative piece published. I think in hearing both of you talk today, I'm going to need to step away from blogging a little if I want to keep the narrative medicine going.

The first piece I ever published—"Fallibility/Forgiveness"—was about a medical error I made as a first-year resident. Even now, it's hard for me to put into words why I wanted to publish that story. I wrote it to process the terrible things that happened, the guilt I felt about what happened. After I wrote it all down, I looked at it, and in some place inside me, I said, *Hmmm, I wonder if this is worth trying to share with anybody*. And I probably shared it with one or both of you. I don't know what it is about one particular story that makes me think I should show it to somebody to see if anything comes from it.

The only story I can think of, the one I knew I wanted to do something with after writing the first draft, was the piece on my colleague's suicide. I was compelled to do something with my unrelenting anger and frustration about this silent epidemic of physicians who commit suicide every year.

It's hard for me to say if I have a favorite story. They are all so personal that I feel I'm going to take something away from one of them if I don't mention it.

JOEL: You both focused on the first piece you had published, and that's the way I feel also. It's been so long that I have no idea why I did this initially. Jon said it's the actual pressure, the need to write, and I think we're not being totally honest if we don't include thinking about getting published. I'm just saying that it's nice to get some recognition and see your name in print, and having people say, "Oh, I liked that," or "I cried when I read that," has something to do with it—at least for me it does. But I think that's still not enough, and there must be some other reason why we write—because we're also exposing ourselves, even risking the fact that people will say, "Why in the world did you write that? What were you thinking?" Maybe that's another reason we want to take risks: we want to expose ourselves and see what happens.

JEN: I think you're alluding to the validation we get from colleagues, even if we don't know them personally. I think it does my ego good. When you see that someone responds to your piece—how you interpreted the story, what your role was, how others identify with the emotions you felt—it is very validating.

JOEL: I was going to talk about the first story I published. I think besides the fame we talked about, I was becoming comfortable with myself as a doctor and I had reached a point where I was not as worried about knowing things as much as I could. I was becoming competent in taking care of people, and I wanted to share that in writing. That brings up another thought that we might talk about: Do you think writing stories makes you a better doctor or takes away from being a good doctor? What effect does writing have on you as a doctor?

JON: I don't know how much it makes me a better doctor, but writing sharpens my skills at least because I think to be a decent writer, you have to be a good observer and be aware of details and how to put things together in different ways. I think those are similar skills that get sharper as the process of becoming a physician and going through medical school and training occurs. I enjoy people and caring for people. I think those skills of observation and communication and listening are all cornerstones of being a decent writer. I guess they reinforce each other. That was pretty long-winded!

JEN: I agree with you, Jon. I'm not sure writing stories makes me a better doctor directly, but I think processing and deeply thinking about things that have happened to me is valuable. Instead of having all that unprocessed stuff jumbled inside me all the time, carrying it like baggage from patient to patient, I have a catharsis from processing and writing about it. I can then attack the next challenge, whatever it is, a little more freshly than I might have otherwise. When I say that, it makes me wonder why most doctors don't write all this stuff down. The docs who don't write must have some other way to process and maintain their balance. For me, writing definitely does that.

JOEL: I'm not sure it makes you a better doctor, but I think, as Jon says, the skills that are involved in writing are good skills to have as a practicing physician—the observation and the idea that this is another human being you're dealing with and not just someone who's carrying a disease. I think that being able to use these skills for the other is valuable, and I agree, Jen, that there are people who don't write and just don't have the need to put it down on paper.

JON: I think there was a novelist who said the point of writing for him was to connect, so I guess that's what we're doing as writers and as doctors.

JOEL: Do you share your stories with the people you write about? Maybe there's no one right answer for that.

JON: I actually have with several people, and they were all very appreciative. I think they also felt they were being heard not only by me but by a bigger audience. It reminds me of a story I read by Abraham Verghese. He once wrote a case report about a patient of his with AIDS, and when he showed it to the patient and was studying the patient's face as he read the story, he could tell the patient was getting kind of upset. So he asked, "What's wrong?" The patient said, "Well, I knew you were going to write a story about me, but this isn't a story about me at all." Verghese had written a very medical, terminology-laden case report, and it was disappointing to the patient because he wanted Verghese to tell his human story, not the story of his liver enzymes and X-ray reports.

JOEL: It's a story and a clinical report.

JON: Yes.

JOEL: My experience is always to share what I've written with the patient or patient's family before actually getting a final OK to publish it. I think some of the journals require it. If you're writing a story that involves people, you have to make it anonymous, not use a name, and you have to get permission from the patient. I think I've always done that, and almost all the time people are very happy that you took the time and energy and the thought to write about them. I can't ever recall anyone saying "That's not me," or "You got it wrong."

Jen, what's your experience and how do you handle it?

JEN: I don't think I have directly shared anything I've written with a patient or a family. I think part of this is because a couple of the experiences I've had were with patients and families whom I only cared for one day or one night when I was a resident on call. When I initially wrote these stories, again, the plan was not to publish them. When I decided to try and publish a couple of them, I changed names and details to preserve anonymity.

In "Our Family Doctor," I tell the story of a patient of mine who died during my second year of residency; his wife and I made the decision together to withdraw him from aggressive medical care. I did mention to her a year or two later that I had written about him and she seemed to think that was very nice, but I don't remember asking her if she wanted to see it. I think, partly, I was afraid of having her see it because she had a really prolonged grief reaction after his death. I was nervous that my emotional account of that time might make things worse for her. Maybe, in retrospect, I should not have been so egotistical as to think that reading my story could have had that big an effect on her. Maybe it would have been healing for her—but she never asked and I never offered.

JOEL: Bringing up our own needs, do either of you see any danger in writing these stories? Do they become ours and become possessed by us, or are we in some way taking the story away from the patient by writing, publishing, and sharing it?

JEN: I don't think so. I think that especially in the blogging world, there are a lot of patients' voices out there—and I think patients are being heard in a way they never have before. So I don't think so. One of the things that can be challenging, which I alluded to earlier, is respecting patients' privacy. When you publish a story in a journal, you change a few details. The only other people who are probably going to see that journal article are medical types.

In the blogging world, you have no editor. You just say what you want, hit a button, and it goes online. There have been docs who have gotten into a lot of trouble because they've written unkind things about patients. They didn't do a very good job of disguising who their patients were; their patients found out about it; and consequences like lawsuits, job loss, and sanctions ensued.

In the blogging world, there's a hot debate now among physician bloggers about whether it's OK to tell personal stories about patients. Some argue you should just stick to generalities in medicine. I'm kind of on the fence about that one because I see the risks. Anyone can find what you write on the Internet. It can be tempting to put things out there that might not be construed as being professional. Somehow, on the Internet you can be even more personal than most journal editors would let you be.

At the same time, I don't want to see storytelling go away. As things get more and more digital, as we move more and more away from print, I'm hoping there's still going to be a place for us to tell a patient's story and feel safe in doing that—because now there's definitely a sense among most physician bloggers that it's not safe to tell stories about individual patients unless you explicitly get permission.

JOEL: I've read some books written by psychiatrists who tell a lot of stories that you would think made the patient more identifiable. Certainly, when we're writing our stories, we try not to use real names, and we alter a story enough so that you can't identify the patient. But that's not perfect either. You have to be concerned because you don't know what the effect is going to be on the people who read their story.

JEN: Absolutely.

JON: I think when you write for a peer-reviewed journal, Joel, you have editors who are very experienced, who are pretty good at guiding you. I have learned how to write with the help of many editors, and they really put a premium on not trying to be gratuitous—in the use of the patient experience, anyway. That's very valuable, because a lot of times we do write about very difficult, stressful, depressing subjects. Then the story we write comes down to what we've learned and what we hope other people will connect with or get something out of, and we have to be careful and respectful about not taking advantage of our situation as doctors who have this very intimate context with our patients.

So Jen, in that sense, it's a very good point you make about blogging. You can be pretty emotional and pretty immediate, and you can just get something out there without having an editor telling you to take a step back—though you may need that many times. I think you need to be careful with that or a little more thoughtful sometimes.

JOEL: This conversation reminds me of our prior discussion about generational differences. I tried to write about long-term relationships, but as Jen pointed out, many of your stories—since you started at a younger age—are about briefer encounters that were powerful and worth sharing. Though when you write about long-term relationships, it's hard to be anonymous. There are too many stories that duplicate each other. If you write about patients you've been with thirty years, it's up to them to figure out who they are.

JON: Right.

JEN: So I have to interrupt you, Joel. I'm really struck by the fact that we're talking about some really difficult things, and Jon made a comment that the bulk of the things that we write about are not happy things. There's not too much that we have written about where we celebrate our successes, although the successes are also why I love family medicine—and I'm sure all three of us have lots of those stories to tell.

JON: I joked before that if we were writing happy things, we would be writing songs instead of stories. But I think these difficult stories are more interesting—well, that's my bias because stories like this show conflict or drama.

JOEL: Well, country music songs are all very sad.

JON: That's true: "Someone done somebody wrong."

JEN: Are we too self-deprecating to write about our successes? Do we fear that we're not going to be viewed as humble, or are success stories truly not worth writing?

JOEL: If you read the stories that are published in medical journals, some have happy endings and sometimes I feel that the writer is trying to make himself feel good and pat himself on the back. I think maybe those stories are doing what the three of us are hoping we should do. What we should be doing is writing about good things, about why it's so wonderful to be a doctor and live this kind of life.

JON: Plus, maybe the kind of media that we write through, as it evolves, will change what we write about in some way. Jen, I've noticed that when you write in your blog, you deal with topics like making mistakes or grief, about technology and electronic health records. Blogging seems to be an easier and maybe more expeditious way to write about things that make you happy or interested. You can just get it out, so that people will digest your words quickly rather than looking for that thing that's going to be too thought provoking, heavy, or profound.

JEN: That's true. The blogs that I read or follow the most are not super-thought-provoking treatises, and the folks who write these blogs do good work. Some of those blogs are well written and describe important ideas, but I find those are not the ones I gravitate to most of the time. When I'm reading the blogs, I want something that is interesting and thought provoking, that's easy to read, and that gives me that sense of "OK, I got my little moment. Next!" I guess my expectations are lower.

JOEL: In thinking about the few stories I've written and the many I've read, I think maybe we're wrong, that they're not all so sad. A lot of these stories are about people dying, but they're usually about a good patient-doctor relationship and how the doctor helped, and I think many of them are celebrations of being a doctor and the powerful relationship that develops between doctor and patient. Just because someone dies in the story does not mean that it is totally a sad story.

JEN: That's true.

JON: I think for the writer, the purposes of the story would be to show that life goes on no matter what the ending is, that someone learns from the story (presumably the storyteller), and that there are things worth celebrating.

JOEL: It strikes me that these stories are so popular with everybody, particularly the doctors who read them, and yet it's hard to find the people who practice the way it's described in the story. I'm not sure what the barriers are, but many doctors seem to admire these stores but not emulate them.

JON: Isn't that human nature?

JOEL: I'm really being unfair, because I really don't know how people live or practice.

JEN: It's the same thing that comes up while I sit on all these electronic health record committees. People don't like responding to the "best practice alerts" because they interrupt their workflow, and physicians say to themselves, "Yeah, if I had all the time in the world, of course I would do all that health maintenance and all that preventative stuff—but I don't. I have this busy real-world practice and I don't have time."

Well, I guess I'm still young and naïve enough to believe that there really *is* time to do all that and have a relationship with a patient.

Making Mistakes
and the Dark Side
of Medicine

JOEL: Jen, one of the topics you wrote about was whether you had committed malpractice, whether you would be sued. I think sometimes we don't pay enough attention to doctors' feelings about this difficult situation, although there is a lot written about malpractice and how to improve care. But there are so many more situations in which the doctor worries about malpractice or blames himself or herself for something that went wrong. Maybe we should talk a little bit about those feelings rather than the "usual" topics related to making mistakes.

JEN: I must admit that my story "Fallibility/Forgiveness" was about my fear that I would be sued. However, after I talked to the attending about my patient's presentation and described how ill this gentleman already was with his cancer, that fear went away. But that fear was nothing in proportion to—and I don't know what the right word is because "guilt" does not seem strong enough—that moral realization that I had ended this man's life.

JOEL: When I published my story with the title "Malpractice?" the editor asked me to change the title because I had originally written the word *malpractice* with several question marks after it. I wrote him back and said that the whole point of the story was highlighted by the question marks, because there are a lot of times when things go wrong and nobody else but the doctor asks, "Did I do something wrong?" And I think that's what was going through my head there. Obviously, the situation bothered me so much that I believed things had happened that didn't happen, and I thought I saw things in the chart that were not there, and ultimately there was no malpractice suit.

However, that doesn't mean there was no malpractice. I think we all find ways to blame ourselves for things—like you described in your story, Jen—but I know now that I didn't do anything wrong in the story I wrote. That doesn't stop us from blaming ourselves, whether we call it malpractice or not; we feel responsible and we feel that we have done something that was not ideal practice.

JEN: I almost wish there was another term for what happens besides *malpractice*, because I feel that word is so wrapped up in thoughts of law, lawyers, money, and courtrooms, and I don't think those connotations get to the heart of how we as physicians really feel about it.

JON: I agree, it's how you define malpractice because I think the word has all those other meanings concerning the legal aspects, your licensure, and losing money and your reputation. But malpractice is still in that continuum of making mistakes, so when we talk about how we deal with ourselves when we make mistakes, we look over our own shoulders realizing other people are looking over our shoulders too. We are our own harshest critics, and this is one of the attributes that's good about how we are as family doctors—or any kind of physician—but it also causes us to be hardest on ourselves.

JEN: My least favorite part of being a physician is thinking about the possibility of making a mistake. I wish I could do what I do all day long and not have to worry if I made the right or wrong choice.

JOEL: In other words, if you could be perfect.

JEN: Joel, I envy you in your retirement. You don't have to go home every night and worry, "Did I miss something?" or "What mistake did I make?"

JOEL: Before I retired, I would bump into people my age who were already retired and my question would always be "What is retirement like; how is it?" The most consistent answer I got was "No responsibility." That was the most important thing. It was not the free time, it was not playing golf or doing what they wanted to do; it was giving up responsibility, because there is so much responsibility in the work we do.

JEN: I think it's hard for folks who are not physicians to really grasp how deep it is for us. I think my family members and other non-physicians are certainly empathic listeners, but I don't know if you truly understand how deep that responsibility is without living it. I think your story, Joel, effectively describes the heaviness of that feeling. You make very real the emotions that you were experiencing then.

JOEL: I think that fear of malpractice adds to that. It's not the cause, it's not the most important thing, but it does add. As I said in the story, I felt that I did something wrong—and I constantly worried that I was going to be punished, my reputation was going to be ruined, my money was going to be taken away, and I wasn't going to be able to take care of my family. But on the other hand, even without the threat of malpractice we would still be berating ourselves.

JON: We definitely are our own harshest critics. Joel, here's how you poignantly described it: "I did not hear from the family, which only heightened my concerns; I began sleeping poorly, waking often, usually from an unremembered but horrible dream;

I fretted and obsessed during my waking hours as well, whether at work or with my family." It's so accurate. I can really relate to those feelings. I think of things I've done or worried that I did or didn't do, which made me just as vulnerable.

JOEL: Jon, someone that I respect read "Malpractice?" before it was published and loved the last sentence. Can you read it?

JON: I'll read the end of the piece:
"There is a two-year statute of limitations on malpractice suits in Pennsylvania. I slept better and functioned better during the rest of those two years. I always expected that accusing letter to come, but it never did, and when the last day came and went, I felt shocked and exuberant.

"But I felt sad and incomplete that I never saw anyone in that family again."

JOEL: So it's not just the fear of malpractice. Of equal importance is what harm you do to yourself and also the implications about severed relationships—because I never saw anybody in that family again.

JON: The piece I wrote set in Alaska called "Procedure Note" was about several mistakes I made in the course of a busy day, and one of the issues I briefly raised in the story was malpractice. I mentioned malpractice in the context of how we write our medical notes, trying to be thorough and comprehensive and very professional—how we write notes this way not only for ourselves but also for the benefit of the attorneys who might be reading them in the future.

It's an unusual dilemma, one that creates such a weird social environment for us as doctors. On the one hand we're trying to be empathic and sincere, to establish rapport with a patient so he or she trusts us and likes us. Then the person leaves the room and we write these very dry, clinical notes sounding like we're scientists who've just observed a very objective set of facts and as if we're just cold, objective persons.

However, we're really using all our senses, trying to be good people and good clinicians. I think one reason we write notes this way is to satisfy the science of medicine and yet also satisfy attorneys who are looking at the things we missed and didn't do. This writing style reflects the very stressful dual life we lead as professionals. As Jen was saying earlier, it's hard for people who aren't in medicine to relate to that. We're trying to be honest and also avoid getting sued, and it's just this dance that is very energy consuming.

JOEL: Although this is not directly related to malpractice, it is interesting that while the three of us write stories, Jon is saying that when we write our clinical notes we're not writing a story. Over the years, many physicians—such as Rita Charon, who has taught and advocated for narrative medicine—have said that physicians may simply be too busy in their daily care of patients. She says that the ideal way to document patient encounters would to be to write their story as the patient tells it—not with that cold, factual note. Maybe we would even read each other's notes more if there were a story in place of the same cold, clinical words that we always repeat.

JEN: I think there's an art to writing a good progress note, and I'm guilty, as a teacher, of not spending as much time as I should working with students and our residents on this skill. Our biggest challenge in the last few years is the widespread adoption of electronic health records (EHR). Back in my early residency days, we would dictate all the progress notes; you would read these and they were almost narratives. Even if they were filled mostly with objective facts and information, they still had the flow of somebody who was speaking.

However, EHRs allow us to be more time efficient by giving us stock phrases to use for documentation. For instance, you can

213

use the exact same pre-completed physical exam note for every patient. How do you make these prefabricated notes reflect an individual person? We hear a lot of our colleagues with the same complaint now: "Well, this note could have been about anybody—it's just a generic note." I think this kind of documentation will become more widespread now—I predict that dictation is going to quickly fade as the generations who relied on it retire and the folks who are raised on EHR are just typing and "dot phrasing" (using pre-completed stock phrases) and all that other stuff.

JOEL: To me the biggest problem is the implication that these stories have nothing to do with the care of the patient and that all we need is to do is put down the medical facts—when in essence, it's a person who has a disease and we don't write anything down about that person. The story, the person's narrative, tells all about that person as an individual—and we're losing the narrative.

JEN: I would agree with that wholeheartedly, and my own solution for that dilemma is that I'm a very fast typist (although a lot of folks aren't); my prior writing background helped me develop those skills. I type fast enough to free-text my history of present illness (HPI) while the patient is talking, using the patient's own words. I don't use any prewritten text for the patient's history, and I started to do that because I was unhappy with how those notes were looking if I used pre-completed notes. I don't think I could go back to using stock phrases.

JOEL: Fifty years ago, when I was in medical school and they taught us the HPI, the first thing you were supposed to do was to write a personal story, if you will, about each patient, and then go into the chief complaint and the complaints. But first, you described who that person was.

We've gotten a little bit off track, as is supposed to happen in this kind of free-flowing conversation, but one of the things we're all talking about with mistakes and malpractice are the guilt feelings that we all have. Related to these topics, both of you have written more than I have about suicide and the guilt that goes along with that for everybody—not just the doctors but everyone associated with that person. Maybe we can talk a little bit about what you've written as well as what you may not have written.

JEN: Sure, Joel, I can speak to that. The piece "Today I Am Grieving a Physician Suicide" was another essay that definitely started out as something I never intended to publish or share. It was a narrative in which I described what I was feeling, and guilt and grief were the parts that I wrote about first. I added the numbers/statistics and medical literature review later, after I originally submitted that raw, emotional piece to the *Annals of Family Medicine*. Thankfully, an editor there saw the potential in the piece and made some very wise suggestions to add that objective, clinical stuff in.

I think if you have a piece that's nothing but emotion, it's hard to be stirred to do much by that when you've finished reading it. It doesn't sustain itself. But if you can say, "Look, this is happening. It's happening over and over again. Here are the statistics," then this hopefully creates a call to change. That was my goal, and eventually sharing it and getting it published—well, I needed to do something with the anger that persisted past my grief and my guilt.

JON: What about the guilt you had?

JEN: I still have it in some respects, though it has lessened. I have read since then that guilt is a "normal part" of the response after you lose someone to suicide who was a friend or a colleague—or anyone close in your life. It took me a year or more after this death to realize that sometimes, as doctors, we want to be omnipotent—but we're not. We have thoughts like "Well, I can stop this person's hypertension and I can talk this person into getting a flu shot, even though they really don't want it," and similarly, in this case, I kept thinking, "I could have saved my friend from committing suicide." We want to believe we have the power to do those things, but I came to the realization that I probably did not have the power to stop my friend from doing this. That was not a very comforting thought at first because I wanted to believe I did, but this realization of powerlessness is where I uneasily ended up.

Suicide grief is different to me from other grief I've experienced from folks who died from more natural causes. Like any grief, it resurfaces from time to time and can be provoked by completely random things, like songs you remember that you shared with a loved one or any similar experience that just prompts the memory and the grief. But the grief from suicide always comes with an additional layer of . . . I don't know what the word for it is. It's almost sadness above and beyond because it was a premature death and . . . I don't know, I'm sorry, I'm not sure what I'm trying to say. I think there's something else with it.

JOEL: Think about it. I think suicide accentuates the feelings that we all have when someone dies. I would say to patients when there was a death in the family that I have never had someone die without everybody around feeling guilty. Even the people who did the most, did the best job of taking care of that person, always found some way to feel guilty that they could have done more. I think everybody has that, and the doctor has more than his or her share of that. Suicide just multiplies that feelings of guilt and responsibility and reminds us of what we could have done differently.

JEN: That's a good point.

JOEL: I think all people connected to the person who has committed suicide—even people who were not close the situation—try to figure out what they could have done to change the outcome.

JON: I think the guilt part is different from the guilt we have about malpractice and about our own standards of how we as doctors take care of others. I like the way, Jen, you wrote your piece like a letter talking to your friend who killed himself. The letter format highlights the feelings you have when someone commits suicide: you feel like saying "If only I had said something, or if I had known this, or if you knew how I was feeling, or if we had only talked together about this—then maybe this horrible thing would not have happened." So this essay you wrote is really primarily a letter to this person telling him how much you cared for him and expressing this unfulfilled desire that "maybe I could have helped prevent this terrible event just by talking to you."

JOEL: If there had been another chance, I could have made a difference, I could have changed the outcome.

JON: That's right.

JEN: I think this piece, more than anything I've written in my short career, has generated a lot of response—and I still, about every other month or so, will get a random e-mail from someone who googled "physician suicide" because they know somebody who committed suicide or something has happened, and they come across this piece. Sometimes I get these gut-wrenching e-mails about a lost spouse, friend, partner, or whomever. They tell me that they found my piece, and usually there is a thank-you for writing it. But then there's this horrible "I don't know what to do," or "I don't know how I'm feeling," or "Do you think there's something I could have done?" It's as if they're asking me to be a therapist or a confessor.

JON: Or a priest.

JEN: Every time I get one of those e-mails, it's just like somebody has sucker-punched me. The stories are as awful and as emotional as mine or Jon's, and to me, when I get asked to speak about this as I have in other forums (and as I will again in a few months), there's a part of me that wants to say no. I don't want to think about this anymore. I want to close this chapter. It's like someone's picking at an open wound and I say, "It hurts too much, stop!"

But then there's a part of me that still thinks, "Well, if only I could have done one more thing…" So this is my one more thing. I feel I owe it to my friend to say yes because maybe I can help somebody help somebody else—which sounds incredibly naïve and silly as I say it out loud—but that is my motivation, and I continue to stay involved with this topic.

I wish I had never had the opportunity to become a supposed expert on physician suicide. It was not anything that I planned for or wanted in my career, and I still hate it sometimes—but from one piece, it shows the power of narrative writing in medicine. I wrote one piece, and I have talked to other people who talked to other people, and I have been interviewed about this in a few places and participated on panels, and all of a sudden, bam: "You're an expert." I wish I had never had reason to be an expert in this.

JOEL: It's a very painful thing to be an expert on. It seems to me that suicide is the ultimate rejection—that we get angry at people who leave us or who die, but suicide is to purposefully leave, and it just stirs up all kinds of feelings in those of us who feel rejected and also feel responsible.

JEN: Definitely true. Jon, I like your piece. My piece was very selfish, but I like how in your piece you wrote about how you and another colleague heard a survivor's story, and in that way you were supporting the survivor.

JON: Jen, you and I had talked about writing about suicide for several months after going through these two horrible situations within such a short period of time in our residency program. After going through that process that everyone does— the guilt, the anger, the sadness—the process of writing this poem, "Bereavement," was interesting because I wrote a lot of it rather quickly within a few months.

For several months before he died, I had worked alongside the person who had committed suicide and his best friend. Writing this poem was spurred on by working side by side with his best friend for a few years after he died, hearing her story, and watching her go through her own really profound grief. I had written this poem and revised the ending of the poem several times, and this poem was published three or four years after I first started to write it. The ending I wrote initially had to do with feeling lost, without a foundation of belief, and months later I changed it to sound a little bit more benign. Then for some reason, when I finally finished this poem, I gave it more of an optimistic tone.

The *JAMA* editor wrote in her comments that it reminded her of a belief in reincarnation or something like that. When I wrote the ending this way, I didn't think of reincarnation *per se*, but I did think of a phoenix rising out of the ashes, a reemergence of belief or some kind of optimism. And so the poem—how I wrote it over time—was more like a process of how my own thoughts about it happened, about going from grief to despair to finding optimism and belief again. It's such a lengthy process.

Just today, by sheer coincidence, one of the patients I saw in the office was a lady whom I've known for about twelve years, whose grown son committed suicide almost exactly two years ago; this was an unspeakably terrible anniversary. I was seeing her in follow-up; she has been very depressed and grieving the last two years. Although she said the last two weeks had been very difficult and she had been crying more, she has still been able to spend time with her daughters and family to take care of them, and she's trying to walk a lot in her backyard swimming pool.

I have seen slow progress over her two years of dealing with this profound, really unspeakable, unimaginable grief, and she is still able to take care of herself—but it's so difficult. Today she showed me two photos of him—one at a dinner party, where he's smiling and happy, and one where he's on a roller coaster at Kennywood amusement park, smiling and screaming. She told me, "I found these photos, and some of my family members said I shouldn't look at them too much, but I feel like I should."

I felt this was really something important, and I encouraged her to look at these pictures too because they remind her that he had a lot of happiness in his life as well. It's just a process, like storytelling is a process in which we're writing about ourselves, really, in most respects; these stories are about our own grief.

JOEL: Has anyone written about the grief and despair that doctors go through? There is a lot written about grief and despair for people who lose someone and how much different and worse it is with suicide, but what about doctors whose patients commit suicide?

JEN: That's a good question. I'm trying to remember if I've read anything along those lines—Jon and I both wrote more from the perspective of losing a colleague rather than a patient. In researching my piece, I did come across a very old, twenty- or thirty-year-old piece—I think it was in *JAMA*—that a psychiatrist wrote about a physician who was a patient and not a colleague that he was caring for. This psychiatrist was worried that his physician patient would commit suicide. (One of the things that dismayed me when I started doing the literature review for my essay was how old and outdated the studies were.)

But now some folks are doing research in physician suicide that's starting to get a little bit of publicity. Tom Schwenk, MD, who was at the University of Michigan, has done a lot of work in that regard. He provided some information for my piece, and now the American Medical Association is having a three-part webinar about physician suicide that I'm going to be participating in. This is the first time within my memory that the organization has made a big deal about this issue. I am heartened a little to see that this issue, which used to be very taboo to talk about, is now starting to get a little bit of traction.

Transitions: Saying Goodbye

JON: It has been fun listening to the two of you talking about leaving. However, Jen, your leaving our residency program faculty will be so difficult because we're all going to miss you—and because, as you were saying, it's been so emotional and difficult to have your patients saying good-bye because they're going through their own grieving process now. I was curious about that in terms of your own experiences. Joel has written about retiring and leaving his patients, so I was hoping you could talk a little bit about what you're going through right now.

JEN: I certainly won't pretend to say that my experience is anything approaching the scale of Joel's retirement. I've been with my patients for a little over eight years—not an insignificant amount of time, but not a whole career either. But leaving them is a very difficult process, and one of the things that tells me it's difficult is that as somebody who likes to write about things, I can't seem to write about it yet. This experience is still so raw. I've done a few blog entries about leaving and about transition, hoping that the blog will serve as a record of that process. Maybe for other folks who are going through a transition like this, the blog will serve as a sounding board, a reflection; I've looked for sources like that myself and haven't found them. There's not a lot of writing about what it's like to transition to a new place as a physician.

It's hard. These patients, many of whom have given me so much enjoyment in our relationships—through getting to know them, celebrating their successes, and even grieving their losses during the years—have all given me so much. And yet they're now coming in for appointments to say good-bye to me with cards, letters, and little tokens of thanks. It's so completely overwhelming for me I don't even know how to process it.

I told one of the staff members after my office session this morning that I've just given up any thought on running on time until I leave because you just cannot rush those good-byes. I was running forty-five minutes behind by the time I finished my morning session today. Every single person on my schedule came in, and we spent a lot of time reminiscing—and maybe not spending so much time doing "medicine."

Then one of the staff members said, "Oh goodness, you've been with them for a long time, of course you deserve that." I bristled at that word *deserve*, because I was really just doing my job. And I thought back to the statement I've heard you say, Joel, that our greatest healing potential as physicians is in the relationship—not in the things we prescribe and other things that we do. I had always thought that maybe someday, I would be that doctor who was able to use myself as the most powerful instrument for my patients. This morning I had this realization that, at the risk of not sounding humble, maybe I was that for some of these folks a little bit.

JOEL: I'm sure you were.

JEN: I always feel when folks are generous to me that it's more a reflection of their generosity and goodness than anything I've done, and I feel that very strongly about the things my patients are saying and writing to me as I prepare to leave.

JON: I don't think that's true. I don't think it's that one-sided. I don't think they would be responding to you like that if they didn't feel that you were the person that was giving them so much.

JEN: I appreciate that, Jon. It's interesting because we've talked a lot about mistakes and guilt and asking ourselves the question, "Did I do the right thing?" I've done a lot of that with my patients over the last eight years. I wish I could say that I do less of it now that I'm an attending. When I first got here as an intern, I experienced all the worrying, asking myself "Did I do the right thing with this medicine? Did I order the right test? Was it OK to watch this or should I have followed up on that?" But for all the agonizing, what my patients are celebrating is our relationship. They're not saying "I'm glad you sent me for this test," or asking "Did you put me on Zocor?" Nothing like that.

JOEL: Because those clinical decisions and actions are important, but they're not on the same level of importance as your personal and professional relationships with them.

JEN: It's very reassuring to know that it's OK not to be perfect as long as you keep working on that relationship.

JON: As long as you can.

JEN: So there are a lot of disjointed, unprocessed thoughts.

JOEL: What about you, Jon? You've moved a couple of times; you've had to say good-bye more than once.

JON: I felt like I was almost kind of an expert at it for a while.

JOEL: You've been here how long now?

JON: I've been here ten years now, which is the longest I've been anywhere in my life. When I listen to you talk about your upcoming move, Jen, and when I read Joel's eloquent writings about transition, these conversations with your patients are a celebration of your caring, right? Your patients care for you because you cared for them, and like somebody once said, caring is the most important part of the relationship.

I previously worked at a community health center in Boston for seven years, and when I left, the nicest present I got was a photo album the nursing staff had made for me. This album had all these pictures of patients alongside little notes the patients had written, and that was the most wonderful present I ever could have received: to have this photo album and see these faces of these people. It's just a celebration of people, and as corny as it sounds, we are specializing in relationships. In family medicine, that's what we say we do, and we do it well.

JOEL: One of the Academy's mission statements is "Wouldn't you like someone who specialized in you?" That's what we like to think we do, and I think we have to admit it's a good feeling to be liked. We want to be liked—not receive adulation—and one of the things that's so important to us as individuals doing our job is that people do appreciate us and like us. As much as we care for them, they care about us.

JON: That's true.

JOEL: About saying good-bye, I wrote "What Would I Do Without You?" It was after I had heart surgery, and it was really about two opposing things. First, I really appreciated how much people cared and asked about me and worried about me. Second, I realized that my patients would get along without me—although I wasn't sure I would get along without them! It was clear that someone else caring and capable would take care of them, and they would be OK with that—which was good for the patient but at the same time upsetting to me as their physician.

JEN: I agree.

JOEL: We want to feel like we're the only ones who can do this and the only ones who have this special right, but that's not true. It makes you feel good when they say, "You know, there will never be anyone like you."

JEN: Didn't Mr. Rogers say that? Every June, we go through this process where all the graduating residents' patients realize how traumatic it is to say good-bye to their resident primary care physician (PCP). We hear them tell us "This resident was my favorite resident," and "They were so good and I can't bear to have that happen again, so can I have an attending for my PCP now so that they won't leave?" The other attending will say no, and by August the patients are fine with their new resident PCP. So not to minimize the thoughtfulness that goes into all the wonderful things folks say when we leave, but I have to agree with you, Joel—in a few months, they'll be fine.

JOEL: So that realization made me think very clearly about not getting too excited about leaving.

JEN: Like everything else in medicine, there's a balance. You don't want to get too far into feeling that "all my patients love me and I am the greatest doctor ever," but you don't want to downplay the importance of what we do for our patients and the fact that we ourselves are the most potent medicine we have to offer our patients. I've definitely absorbed a lot of that lesson in the last few weeks.

JOEL: I think it's important to accept how important we are and to accept the fact, which is good, that they will get along without us.

JEN: Yes, simultaneously.

Conclusion

We have produced a book that includes our stories and our discussions about the content and meaning of those stories. We believe that medical care depends on listening to patients' stories, determining the meaning of those stories, and using that information for the benefit of our patients. This is not a new idea but one that needs reemphasis with constant vigilance so that doctors think about patients and their stories—not just their diseases or symptoms.

These ideas and examples can be useful in educating medical students and residents not only to improve the care they provide but also to make their work more interesting and challenging. This book can also be of use to patients in encouraging them to tell their story and to expect personal care and attention from their doctor.

Our book is unique in that it includes the experiences and ideas of three family doctors of three different generations. We have found that we have different ways of telling our stories and even different ways of hearing them, but the basic attributes of the doctor-patient relationship remain the same and are dependent on caring and knowing patients as people.

Perhaps the most important thing that happened in this writing collaboration was the reassurance it gave to each of us that there is a better way to care for patients—and that we share that better way over our three generations.

It has been our privilege to share our collective journey as medical writers with you. If you are a physician, we hope that you might also consider sharing your stories and experiences

227

with others—and to this end, the following pages include a list of places you might consider submitting your stories to. After all, as physicians, we will always have so much to learn from one another.

Afterword

By Paul Gross, MD

What I like best about this book—and what makes it so
invigorating—is that it plays against type. This is a book about
family medicine, written by family doctors, and yet their reports
from the field are refreshingly different from one another.

Joel Merenstein's communiqués about small town family
medicine surprise one with their intensely personal tone. How
many doctors express such vulnerability when writing about their
patients? (Are doctors even supposed to do that? some readers
may ask.) I may not have gotten the medicine a hundred percent
right all of the time, he seems to be telling us, but I did get my
relationships with my patients right. And, looking back from the
vantage point of my retirement, that's what really mattered.

Dr. Merenstein's patients get depressed. They say that things
are fine when they really aren't. They worry. They die young. Or
they age and die old. With each loss, our doctor-guide loses a
piece of himself. He cries. And yet he carries on. Family members
reach out to him. Occasionally blame him. And sometimes arrive
on his doorstep as brand-new patients.

I'm as human as my patients, he seems to be telling us.
Their story is my story. We're in this together.

Jonathan Han arrives at family medicine from a vastly
different perspective, that of an outsider—a Korean-American
raised in a Midwestern town where Asians were few and far
between, and in a time when intolerance was the norm. He grew
up being given a hard time for being who he was and looking

the way he looked. His writing is movingly effective: we feel the stings and the threats, and we also marvel at his pointed sense of humor.

Not surprisingly, his journey has informed his practice of medicine. He delivers care to the underserved--who, as it turns out, also give him a hard time, and sometimes for the same reasons his small-town schoolmates did. Yet his patients are underdogs in life's struggle, and by simply being who they are, they win his (and our) compassion and understanding.

Dr. Han also pulls the camera back to ask big questions about our healthcare system. Why does it make impossible demands of him and his residents? (Discharge your hospitalized patients faster! But don't cut corners! And remember: It's your fault if they're readmitted, even for reasons you have no control over!) Why does our system deny care to so many? And why do we tolerate this?

His pieces invite us to care about the patients he introduces us to, and about the patients we will never meet. He asks us to consider our responsibility to our human community.

Jennifer Middleton is another physician who is not afraid to reveal the heart that beats beneath her white coat. She tells us about a colleague who committed suicide; about a patient's death for which she, as a resident, blamed herself; about the first time the mantle of "family doctor" was bestowed upon her--by the wife of a dying patient; and about her own frightening medical diagnosis. These pieces are heartfelt--sometimes heartbreaking.

Then Dr. Middleton takes us into new territory—the field of family medicine itself and its place in the world of medicine. She is an advocate for this quintessential primary-care specialty that provides so much of what patients and communities want and need, as the stories in this book so vividly demonstrate. And yet, alas, most patients don't know what family medicine is. Medical schools often give our specialty short shrift. And our nation's third-party payers value the comprehensive generalist far less than the procedure-minded partialist. So how, exactly, will this nation acquire the primary-care workforce that it so badly needs? Dr. Middleton offers some ideas.

One leaves this book with vivid impressions of these three family physicians, who serve as exemplars of our specialty--and models for the practice of medicine.

Drs. Merenstein, Han and Middleton embody virtues that we all want in our personal physicians: They are open and human. They're not afraid of their vulnerabilities. (On occasion, they'll even wear their hearts on their sleeves.)

They navigate medical science and medical institutions with calm expertise.

They believe in the power of relationships.

They take pride in their work while conducting themselves with humility and humor.

They are advocates--for their patients, for their communities, for the humanity in each of us and for their specialty.

For those of us in family medicine, Drs. Merenstein, Han and Middleton are reminders of why we're here. For those en route to careers in medicine, these three physicians have blazed a human and heroic path that inspires others to follow.

Acknowledgments

We would like to thank the friends and colleagues who have reviewed our manuscript at various stages, often more than once: Larry Cuban, PhD; Jack Coulehan, MD, MPH; Michele Reiss, PhD; Andrea Gordon, MD; Mary Kinsel; John Frey, MD, MPH; Paul Gross, MD; and Larry Bauer, MSW, MEd.

Thanks also to Paula Preisach, the administrative assistant for our fellowship program, who has had multiple roles with this project. She has been our administrator, guide, and organizer, for all of which she possesses outstanding skills and a most pleasant attitude.

Thanks to our editor, Jennifer Read Hawthorne, who led us through this publishing process with a steady, experienced, and patient eye. We needed her vision.

And to Laurie Douglas, who designed and formatted the book. Laurie served as our guide and consultant into the world of self-publishing, in which we would have been lost without her. Her capability and talent are evident just by looking at this book.

Joel Merenstein

My personal thanks and acknowledgement for help in writing this book goes back long before it was even considered. My two closest friends, Larry Cuban and Dave Mazer, have guided, inspired, modeled, and supported my writing. Dr. Cuban, emeritus professor in the School of Education at Stanford University, has been a prolific writer of books, articles, and blogs, as well as a recognized outstanding teacher and guest speaker. His books occupy an entire shelf in my library. He has constantly and unselfishly shared his ideas, reviewed and commented on my writing, and urged me on by asking, what are you writing now?

Dave Mazer was my first guide in writing when he was the Sports Editor for the *Pitt News* and I was one of his reporters. He has always been kind and gentle in his criticism while continuing to support my efforts. Mary Kinsel, married to a family doctor, entered my life after I retired and participated in a writer's workshop at an Osher Lifelong Learning Institute program. She was one of the co-leaders and taught me the basics I missed when learning to be a doctor.

Various students, residents, and fellows had more or different skills than I and taught me what was important and how to tell it while I was teaching them. Likewise, my colleagues in practice and teaching showed me and taught me about the doctor-patient relationship and the essence of caring for the patient. My original partner, Knighton V. Waite, was particularly instrumental in teaching me to care for people instead of focusing on the disease.

My children have all been successful in their professional careers, but most importantly, they have been nice people, caring for family, friends, and strangers. And of course, my wife, Nancy, who has been part of my life story for over sixty years, has made it possible for me to accomplish whatever I have done in my life. She took care of me while I was caring for others.

Jonathan Han

Looking back on this collaboration with Joel and Jen, I am grateful to have had the opportunity to reflect together on the motivations, difficulties, and joys of writing. We share a love of reading as well as writing, and though we may write about different themes, we each have a passion for family medicine, and we each find meaning being involved in the lives of our patients. I owe Joel and Jen so much for providing the energy and determination to create this project—a labor of love—and make it a reality.

I would like to acknowledge two mentors at San Francisco General Hospital who shaped—and continue to strongly influence—my career in family medicine, Denise Rodgers, MD, and George Saba, PhD. Thank you, Denise and George, for leading tirelessly by your example of commitment and concern for family medicine residency training, and for caring about our local and global communities, always emphasizing service to the underprivileged and advocacy to improve our damaged health care system.

I also want to thank so many writers and friends who have supported me during this writing journey, including Paul Gross, Diane Guernsey, David Loxtercamp, Jerry and Eileen Spinelli, Audrey Young, Pauline Chen, Kevin Grumbach, Jeff Borkan, Jim Valek, Susan Obata, Amita Jain, Hugh Forrest, Dan Shefelman, Mike and Rebecca Bainum, Shiva Saboori, Dave Lee, Michael Madonia, George Kikano, Julia Kasdorf, Paul Han, Kathleen Corcoran, Susan Zucker, Betsy Warner, and Ellen Ficklen.

My partners have given me great joy in the day-to-day practice of medicine, including Nil Das, Mary Popovich, Kathy Connolly, Ellen Hafer, Fred Dolgin, Maria Matsuda, Vibha Bhatnagar, Don Middleton, Ted Schaffer, Jim Mercuri, Patty McGuire, Brittany Sphar, Lucas Hill, Rich Bruehlman, Sandy Sauereisen, Ann McGaffey, Gretchen Shelesky, Mary Pat Friedlander, Marianne Koenig, Erin Imler, Patricia Klatt, Karen Moyer, Vince Balestrino, Kim Flecken, Andie Karsh, Paul Larson, Amy Haugh, Robin Rushnock, Alan McNamara, and Augie Provencio, among so many important others.

For the countless blessings our patients, nursing staff, residents, and team members at the Health Centers have given me, thank you.

I owe a debt of gratitude to my professors and mentors at Kenyon College, who first taught me how to write an organized paragraph: Denis Baly, who taught me the importance of research and brevity; Jay Shiro Tashiro, who encouraged me to analyze and communicate issues of race and relationship with confidence; and especially Royal Rhodes, who to this day continues to guide and mentor me in matters of social justice and the poetry of life.

Thanks to my father, James Sun Nam Han, who first connected me to the power of words spoken with passion to a congregation and his family, and eternal thanks to my mother, Dorothy Sang Ye Han, who first connected me to the power of words spoken with love.

Most importantly, thanks to my wife, Marilyn Fitzgerald, my most trusted editor and inspiration, and our children David and Grace, who listen to stories, read patiently, and ask the most important question: Why?

Jennifer Middleton

I defined myself as a writer a long time before I defined myself as a physician, and there was a time when I foolishly thought those identities were mutually exclusive. I am beyond grateful to the canon of medical writers whose work has shown me the falsehood of that belief.

Without Joel, I would not have become a medical teacher or writer. He created an atmosphere safe enough for me to share my first pieces with him. His boundless encouragement and frank feedback have been invaluable, as was his connecting me with Jon's warm enthusiasm and constant support so many years ago. Much of what I aspire daily to be as a family physician I learned from the two of them.

My teachers at UPMC St. Margaret cultivated a mindset where each patient's humanity and dignity is always at the forefront of my practice as a physician. I learned there not only how to think as a physician but also how to think about being a physician.

Acknowledgments

In recent years, Larry Bauer's zeal for my work in social media has helped connect me to many other physician writers. Each of us, it seems, believes that sharing our stories makes the world a better place—both in continually emphasizing the patient as our priority and also in advocating for the importance of family medicine in our nation's health infrastructure.

Sarah Adams, my best friend since childhood, never let me forget my core self during the grueling years of medical school and residency and, in so doing, kept my writer's soul alive during that time.

My husband, David Banas, and family keep me humble and grounded in the best possible sense of both words. Without their unconditional love, I would not have the courage to share my vulnerabilities on the page.

Contributors

Jack C. Coulehan, MD, MPH (Foreword) is Emeritus Professor of Preventive Medicine and Senior Fellow of the Center for Medical Humanities, Compassionate Care, and Bioethics at Stony Brook University. He graduated from St. Vincent College (BA) and the University of Pittsburgh (MD, MPH) and completed residencies in internal medicine and public health at the University of Pennsylvania, Wake Forest University, and the University of Pittsburgh. Until his retirement in 2007, Jack directed the ethics and humanities program at Stony Brook University Medical Center and chaired the ethics case consultation service at University Hospital. He is the author of over two hundred articles and book chapters in the medical literature, ranging in topic from clinical trials of depression treatment in primary care to studies of heart disease among Navajo Indians to essays on medical humanities, professionalism, and the physician-patient relationship. Jack's poems and stories have appeared in major literary magazines and medical journals in the United States, Canada, England, and Australia. In 2012 he received the Nicholas Davies' Award from the American College of Physicians for "outstanding contributions to humanism in medicine."

Paul Gross, MD (Afterword) is assistant professor in the Department of Family and Social Medicine at Albert Einstein College of Medicine/Montefiore Medical Center, where he teaches narrative medicine to residents. His stories about medical practice and family life have appeared in *American Family Physician*, *Journal of Family Practice*, *Hippocrates*, *The Sun*, *Diversions* and *Town*

& Country. He also conducts award-winning writing workshops for medical professionals. He is the Editor-in-Chief of *Pulse: Voices from the Heart of Medicine*.

Beth Frankel Merenstein, PhD ("Three Generations") is a tenured professor in the Department of Sociology at Central Connecticut State University, where she teaches in the areas of race and ethnicity, immigration, urban studies, and advanced research methods. She has extensive experience with qualitative research and interview analysis in particular. Beth is currently overseeing a program evaluation project examining homelessness prevention.

Resources:
Where to Publish Stories Like Ours

Academic Medicine, "Literature and Arts" and "Lessons From our Learners" sections http://journals.lww.com/academicmedicine/pages/default.aspx

American Family Physician, "Close-ups"(patient narratives) www.aafp.org/online/en/home/publications/journals/afp.html

Annals of Family Medicine, "Reflections" www.annfammed.org

Annals of Internal Medicine, "On Doctoring" section www.annals.org

Archives of Family Medicine https://www.clockss.org/clockss/Archives_of_Family_Medicine

Ars Medica: A Journal of Medicine, the Arts, and Humanities www.ars-medica.ca/

Bellevue Literary Review www.blreview.org/

Blood and Thunder, University of Oregon Health Sciences Center http://www.ouhsc.edu/bloodandthunder/

British Medical Journal, "Personal Views" www.bmj.com

Resources

Dermanities, with a broadly defined dermatology slant
www.dermanities.com

Families, Systems and Health
http://www.apa.org/pubs/journals/fsh/

Family Medicine, "Lessons from our Learners" section
www.stfm.org/publications/familymedicine/index.cfm

Global Pulse—international experience narratives
http://www.globalpulsejournal.com

Healing Ministry, "Healing Vignettes" section
www.pnpco.com/pn04000.html

Health Affairs, "Narrative Matters" section
www.healthaffairs.org

Hospital Drive
https://news.med.virginia.edu/hospitaldrive/

JAMA, "A Piece of My Mind," also a medical student section
www.jama.ama-assn.org

Journal of the American Board of Family Practice—"Reflections"
www.jabfm.org

The American Academy of Hospice and Palliative Care Bulletin,
"Staying Soulful: The Arts and Humanities in Palliative and
Hospice Medicine"
http://aahpm.org

Journal of Medical Humanities
http://www.springer.com/us/

Lance
www.thelancet.com

Literature and Medicine (Johns Hopkins)
http://muse.jhu.edu/journals/literature_and_medicine/

Los Angeles Times weekly health section, "In Practice" www.latimes.com/features/health/la-he-practice-sg,0,1151107.storygallery

Medical Encounter, a publication of the American Academy on Communication in Healthcare
www.aachonline.org

Medical Humanities Online
http://mh.bmj.com

The New England Journal of Medicine, "Perspectives"
http://content.nejm.org/

Patient Education and Counseling, "Reflective Practice" section
http://www.elsevier.com

The Pharos
www.alphaomegaalpha.org

Pulse: Voices from the Heart of Medicine
www.pulsemagazine.org

The Sun, a magazine of personal experience
www.thesunmagazine.org

Yale Journal for Humanities in Medicine
http://yjhm.yale.edu

Permissions

(continued from page ii)

"Malpractice?" is reprinted with permission from *Patient Education and Counseling* 74 (2009): 3–4.

"The Doctor-Patient Relationship I" is reprinted with permission from *Family Medicine: Miscellanea* 19, no. 5 (1987): 338, 388.

"The Doctor-Patient Relationship II" is reprinted with permission from *Family Medicine* 21, no 5 (1989): 5, 18.

"The Doctor-Patient Relationship III" is reprinted with permission from *Family Medicine* 23, no. 8 (1991): 577–79.

"A Preceptor's Story" is reprinted with permission from *Family Medicine* 33, no. 5 (2001): 388–89.

"What Will I Do Without You?" is reprinted with permission from *The Journal of the American Medical Association* 288, no 15 (2002): 1823–24.

"The Family Doctor: A View from Retirement" is reprinted with permission from *Journal of Family Practice* 59, no. 12 (2010): 691–94.

"The Kindest Insult" is reprinted with permission from *BMJ: British Medical Journal* 326, no. 7396 (2003): 991, courtesy of BMJ Publishing Group.

"Welcome to the Arctic Circle" is reprinted with permission from *Journal of the American Board of Family Medicine* 17, no. 1 (2004): 78--79.

"Malignant Neglect" is reprinted with permission from *The Journal of the American Medical Association* 294, no 20 (2005): 2546–48.

"Procedure Note" is reprinted with permission from *The Pharos* 31 (2008).

"Serious Side Effects" excerpt is reprinted with permission from *Health Affairs* 28, no. 2 (2009): 533–39.

"Passing the Torch: A Day in the Life of an Attending Physician" is reprinted with permission from *Health Affairs Blog,* February 1, 2012, http://healthaffairs.org/blog/2012/02/01/passing-the-torch-a-day-in-the-life-of-an-attending-physician/

"Calculating Caring: is reprinted with permission from *Health Affairs Blog,* July 21, 2010, http://healthaffairs.org/blog/2010/07/21/calculating-caring/

"Steep Sledding" is reprinted with permission from *Pulse: Voices from the Heart of Medicine,* October 2, 2009; it is also anthologized in *Pulse: Voices From the Heart of Medicine; More Voices—A Second Anthology* (New York: Change in Healthcare Publishing, 2012).

"Minutes" is reprinted with permission from *BMJ Supportive & Palliative Care* 4, no. 104 (2014) http://spcare.bmj.com/cgi/content/full/bmjspcare-2013-000617/

"Bereavement" is reprinted with permission from *The Journal of the American Medical Association* 303, no 11 (2010): 1016.

Permissions

"Today I'm Grieving a Physician Suicide" is reprinted with permission from *The Annals of Family Medicine* 6, no. 3 (2008): 267–69.

"Fallibility/Forgiveness" is reprinted with permission from *Family Medicine* 41, no. 1 (2009): 13–15.

Author Bios

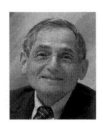 **Joel H. Merenstein, MD,** is Emeritus Director of the University of Pittsburgh Faculty Development Fellowship at UPMC St. Margaret. He is founding Chief of the Division of Family Medicine at the University of Pittsburgh School of Medicine and is presently Clinical Professor in the School of Medicine and Graduate School of Public Health. He maintained a clinical practice in the same community for over 42 years.

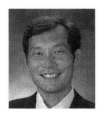 **Jonathan Han, MD,** is Medical Director at UPMC New Kensington Family Health Center, and Associate Program Director of the UPMC St. Margaret Family Medicine Residency Program. After completing his residency at San Francisco General Hospital, Jon worked in a community health center in Boston for several years before moving to Pittsburgh with his family.

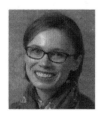 **Jennifer Middleton, MD**, is Associate Director at Riverside Methodist Hospital Family Medicine Residency in Columbus, Ohio. Her residency in family medicine at UPMC St. Margaret was followed by a faculty development fellowship with Dr. Merenstein.

Made in the USA
Middletown, DE
27 January 2017